T0286144

THE
GRIM READER

THE
GRIM
READER

A
Pharmacist's
Guide to Putting
Your Characters
in Peril

MIFFIE SEIDEMAN

RED ⚡ LIGHTNING BOOKS

This book is a publication of

Red Lightning Books
1320 East 10th Street
Bloomington, Indiana 47405 USA

redlightningbooks.com

© 2023 by Mary F. Seideman

Manufactured in the United States of America

First printing 2023

Cataloging information is available from the Library of Congress.

ISBN 978-1-68435-214-2 (paperback)
ISBN 978-1-68435-216-6 (ebook)

The content of this book is for informational purposes only and does not constitute any health or medical advice. The content of this book is not intended to endorse, facilitate, or condone illegal or illicit drug use. Please consult with your own physician or healthcare specialist regarding the health effects of any substances referenced in this book.

For Russ, Tina, and Travis with my unending love and thanks

CONTENTS

PREFACE

Ever had a really bad week and decided to take it out on one of your fictional characters by killing them off with a slow-acting drug? Or were you innocently writing when a character suddenly surprised you by overdosing? Writing these plot twists can be exhilarating, frightening—yes, even therapeutic—adding creative depth to your novel. But if your spy slaps a drug patch onto a character who instantly passes out, or a meth overdose scene ends with a stomach pumped in the emergency room, you risk losing readers.

Since for many authors, the knowledge to write drug-related scenes comes mostly from news headlines or movies, not personal experience, what's written may be more fiction than fact. Some readers may be duped by this, but many are quite savvy. For nurses, doctors, paramedics, family members of those suffering with addiction, or today's worldly young adults, these grossly inaccurate scenes may have gotten you an eye roll followed by a book closure and negative reviews. The same holds true for screenwriters. One adaptation of a poorly researched script led to a show episode depicting surgery with no anesthesia or pain medication, supposedly due to the patient's fear of opioid addiction. There were so many things medically wrong with this concept that the show took a social media beating.

As authors, we spend countless hours writing character arcs, intertwining themes, and painting our canvas with the richness of our imagination. The last thing we want is to lose credibility with our hard-earned readers. Even so, I've seen stories misrepresent drugs, including how they're given, their symptoms, and how fast effects occur. Authors are often intrigued by the idea of a drug that can instantly kill but not be detected during an autopsy. As a pharmacist, I can tell you *that does not exist.* More importantly, this oft-used trope ignores the gift that a real drug timeline offers: time to spin a page-turning scene while the reader's anticipation for the inevitable danger grows.

So, how can you convincingly write a scene involving a teen accidentally using fentanyl-tainted pot or a suicide attempt with Mom's pain pills without a medical background or savvy?

It really isn't hard, given a few key concepts.

With that in mind, this handbook was designed to help authors develop plausible drug scenarios by providing:

- Pertinent drug facts, tips, and symptoms
- Symptom timelines
- Common street drug names and slang
- Sample scenarios to demonstrate how to weave the information into a believable scene
- Writing prompts to provide scene starters and offer practice

Ready to get started? Chapter 1 frames some key facts to consider before you begin writing.

Happy Plotting!

ACKNOWLEDGMENTS

Writing this book meant so much to me. In my last few years of work, it helped me feel valuable in my knowledge, and in my early years of retirement, it has given me purpose. I loved (or hated) writing this book, and I cannot even begin to express how grateful I am to the people who have supported me throughout this multiyear tumultuous journey. There've been so many opportunities for me to fail, and while on some level my inner ego would love to take credit for it all, the reality is that I could not have made it through without my supporting cast, who truly made this production come together in the end.

First, to my husband Russ: I'm not sure that I would've even started this project without knowing that I had your support. From listening to me talk endlessly about my ideas to tolerating me disappearing at a coffee shop—only to come home flustered over my book that I'm sure seemed to you to never make progress—to playing both of our roles at home in the final stretch before publication, your care and devotion shone through. It's not the least bit dramatic to say that the reason I married you was on display through every step of writing this book.

Second, to my agent Amy Collins of Talcott Notch Literary Services: I know this book is an oddball, but I'm so grateful you took it on as a concept. I appreciate your help, support, and tenacity. You were the final piece to the puzzle that I needed to make it all come together in the end.

Third, to my daughter, Tina, and son, Travis: There are no words to describe the amazing support you have both given me from the first moment I had the concept for this book. You've given me the hugs and assurances this monumental task could be done when I needed them, and spent countless hours reading, critiquing, and gently offering what I needed to hear to make this book a reality.

Fourth, to countless others who helped me, supported me, and cheered me to this moment: I'm so utterly grateful to have you in my life.

THE
GRIM READER

1

FIRST THINGS FIRST

Writers have asked how they can realistically describe a drug they've never personally used. How can they accurately portray a character's actions or symptoms? Keep in mind that to sound authentic, scene details don't need to be perfect, but there are a few drug-specific facts, discussed below, that should be right.

Historical Timelines

Building a credible scene requires researching a few historical facts, including:

Was the drug discovered yet?

A scene using insulin set in 1820 is problematic since this treatment wasn't discovered until the 1900s. Fentanyl shouldn't be used in a 1930s scene since it wasn't available for use until the 1960s—opium or morphine would be more accurate choices.

Was the method to take the drug invented yet?

Since insulin must be given as a shot, that scene is even less authentic as the hypodermic needle wasn't invented until the mid-1800s. Older historical fiction could involve the use of poultices and mustard packs, while skin drug patches (transdermal patches) are only appropriate in more modern scenes.

What drug trends existed in the time period of your story?

> *Prescribing trends.* Medical knowledge changes over time and with it the drugs prescribed. This, in turn, impacts the type of prescription drugs diverted into street supplies or available in home medicine cabinets.

Sample Scene #1 He picked up the empty glass vial next to her lifeless body. Chloral hydrate! He'd been a fool to leave it where she could find it.

Is this author's sedative choice realistic? It depends on what year the scene takes place. Popular sedatives have changed significantly over the decades (see chapter 14). In the late 1800s, chloral hydrate was popularly used to treat anxiety and insomnia. It was replaced by bromides, which were also unfortunately used to create the "bromide sleep" to sedate patients in asylums. By the 1920s, awareness that bromides caused prolonged hallucinations led doctors to prescribe barbiturates like phenobarbital (barbital) instead. So, it was no accident that Agatha Christie chose to weave barbital into the plot of *Murder on the Orient Express*. Once the medical profession realized the growing trend of barbiturate addiction, benzodiazepines ("benzos") became the new alternative. Surprisingly, despite safety concerns, it wasn't until the early 2000s that chloral hydrate was finally removed from the US market.

Based on these prescribing changes over time, how would you revise the sample scene to take place in the 1940s? In 2000?

Sample Scene #2 (setting 2020) He quietly opened her medicine cabinet, fumbling through bottles, until his fingers landed on the one labeled "Vicodin."

Writing opiate scenes like this is a great example of how prescribing changes can impact realistic scene choices. Over the last decade, the growing opioid crisis has caused concerns about overprescribing and addiction. But in the early 2000s, poorly treated pain created a national push for better pain control, resulting in increased prescribing of opioid drugs such as oxycodone, hydrocodone (Vicodin), and Percocet. Eventually, this led to an oversupply of opioids, excess stores in medicine cabinets, and increased street supplies. Then, with addiction and overdoses escalating rapidly, additional prescribing restrictions enacted in the US reduced drug availability. The unintended consequence of this was an increase in the black market demand for opioids, which escalated illicit drug smuggling into the US. This influx of opioids has included illicit fentanyl, both in bulk and laced into street drugs such as heroin and counterfeit pain pills. The culmination of these events has resulted in the current fentanyl overdose epidemic. Due to these rapid social changes in a span of only twenty years, an opioid scene set in 2020 will look very different than one set in 2000.

So, is Sample Scene #2 appropriate? If the character's grandmother held onto leftover hydrocodone (Vicodin) after her last surgery a couple of years ago, then yes. Many people, especially the elderly, squirrel away leftover tablets instead of tossing them into the garbage. Some patients hoard pills, afraid they won't be prescribed enough the next time they're in pain.

If the character's grandmother is depicted as having been given the pills after a recent surgery, then no. Opiate prescribing in the US has been extremely restricted during the last several years. Few opioids are prescribed after surgery and when they are, the number of tablets is usually enough for only a few days of treatment. In this case, it would be more realistic to have the character not find the pills he wants and resort to buying some from his friend at school. And where would his friend have gotten the pills? He probably bought them from a stranger at a party. *Now,* how would you finish the scene?

Drug abuse trends. Different countries, and different locations within countries, have varying trends of drug use and abuse over time. Factors affecting these differences are complex, but include laws, local cultures, drug availability, drug costs, and proximity to country borders. A drug-related scene in a town along the US-Mexico border will look quite different than one set in a Midwest farming town. The Resources page at the Drug Enforcement Administration (DEA) website (https://dea.gov/resources) contains a wealth of information regarding location-based trends in drug abuse and even maps of the locations where clandestine labs have been found. *The National Drug Threat Assessment,* published regularly on the site, details national data related to illicit drugs. For international information, a great resource is the United Nations Office on Drugs and Crime website (https://dataunodc.un.org).

Slang terminology. How your character talks about drugs and the related paraphernalia is just as important to sounding authentic as *what* the character does with them. A well-written scene using drug jargon can immerse readers in the setting, even if they don't know what the exact terms mean. A great example of this was developed in the script for the show *Good Girls* (season 1, episode 6) when Boomer pressures Darren into selling him drugs. Darren's response—the litany of drugs he has available to sell, including everything from "Addys" to "fat bags of herb"—is both authentic and funny.

Importantly, drug jargon not only changes over time but also with geographic location, age, socioeconomic status, and a host of other factors. Hundreds of street names and a wide variety of related slang exist for various drugs. A representative sample list of street drug names and slang terms is included in the drug chapters. But applying slang to your scene will require additional research to identify the terms that will sound the most authentic in your story. For example, while *doobie* and *vape* are slang terms used for marijuana, having your 2020s high schooler talk about "takin' a hit off a doobie" would be as out of place as having a 1960s hippie invite someone to "vape some dank weed." And jargon like *dubsack* and *trippin' balls* should be used in the right context.

Online videos posted by recovered drug addicts or current users offer a well-rounded sense of how to apply a broad range of jargon to realistic dialogue. Using the search words *trip report* with the name of a drug or the drug jargon listed in the individual drug chapters is a good starting place to enhance your research. For example, a search for *DXM*, *third plateau*, and *trip report* will result in numerous videos of users that were filmed during their DXM trips, offering profound insight for writing a scene. In addition, a few social influencers have posted videos documenting their journey through drug addiction, recovery, and sometimes even relapse.

Socioeconomic Status

Consider your character's income and the economics of the scene setting. Crack is a credible choice in a plot involving a low-income character because it's a relatively cheap drug, while a cheese platter spiked with ecstasy is more appropriate in a high-society women's brunch scene. Is your character a penniless alcoholic? Instead of passing out after chugging a fifth of Tanqueray gin, the medical responders should find him near death from drinking cheap isopropyl (rubbing) alcohol (see chapter 4).

The market cost of drugs has an impact on drug trends. For example, in about 2013 Arizona high school students switched from abusing expensive oxycodone pills to cheaper and more available heroin. But an influx of illicit pills from Mexico has driven oxycodone prices down, making it the preferred choice again. Many of these pills, however, are counterfeit and tainted with potentially lethal doses of fentanyl. Now, an upsurge of fentanyl overdoses and deaths are being reported in those same high schools (see "Fentanyl" in chapter 13).

DRUG FACTS

How is the drug usually used?

Avoid the temptation to improvise ways to get the drug into your character just to fit a scene. Most drugs given the wrong way won't work as planned. If your villain spikes a drink with insulin to kill an adversary, he'll be sorely disappointed when his victim lives. Insulin must be injected or, in some cases, inhaled, to avoid destruction during digestion.

How fast should a character show symptoms?

Avoid writing instant drug effects. Those scenes are shocking, dramatic, and almost always unrealistic. Instead, build page-turning tension using the actual time it takes for drugs to cause harrowing symptoms. Despite what movies would have you believe, a chloroform-soaked rag won't make a character instantly pass out, and the effects will wear off quickly after the rag is removed. Even injecting drugs rarely works instantly. For example, a villain attempting to kill with an overdose of insulin shouldn't see the victim immediately fall to the ground. Insulin takes time to work, initially dropping the person's blood sugar, leaving his brain foggy, his vision blurry and making him shaky. As his blood sugar drops dangerously low, he can suffer a seizure and lose consciousness. *Now* your character is on the way to dying.

The "he instantly dropped dead" scene is always wrong.

Use the reader's own knowledge and need for suspense to your advantage. Did your character swallow a handful of pills? Since many people know it takes several minutes for pills to have an effect, you can let your readers build their own anticipation, waiting for the inevitable, while you slowly develop the scene tension.

Need to hasten a character's demise? Write the scene using a drug that can be injected into a vein (IV) or inhaled, which generally works faster than a shot into muscle (IM) or swallowed pills. Reserve plots using a skin patch for slow-moving scenes since it takes time for drugs to absorb and cause symptoms. High or lethal doses can rapidly create dangers for your character. But, for *any* of these methods, symptoms should still appear in a cascade, not all at once. For example, a rapid injection of a high fentanyl dose can suddenly cause chest muscles to become rigid, making it hard

Hasten or slow down a character's demise by changing how the drug is taken.

or impossible to breathe. Then, with no oxygen, several other symptoms can evolve—such as blue lips, seizures, a slowing heartbeat, and death—over several minutes (or pages). The character shouldn't die instantly, even with this potent drug.

And keep in mind that not all overdoses are lethal. Depending on the drug, your character may suffer serious symptoms but realistically survive. This fact offers a world of harrowing conflicts that can make your character strong enough to ultimately tackle his inner demons.

What symptoms will the character have?

Your character should have at least a few hallmark symptoms that are typical of the drug. These are listed in the individual drug chapters and the toxidrome tables. Keep in mind, it's important to *not* give your character every symptom to avoid sounding like a checklist. To maintain integrity as a writer, it's also important to not invent symptoms. For example, a scene where your character—who's having an allergic reaction to peanuts—is rescued with an EpiPen (epinephrine auto-injector) *is* realistic. But having a bad guy use an EpiPen to cause a sudden heart attack in your protagonist is *not*.

What's the character's age?

A person's age impacts which drugs are prescribed or abused. Your character's grandparent may have sleeping pills lying around the house, while a high school teen is more likely to have marijuana, oxycodone, or even heroin hidden in his room. Elderly people have more intense side effects, such as confusion, offering interesting twists. In overdoses involving younger children, it's common for a single drug to be involved. So, creating a scene where the emergency room doctor discovers *several* drugs in the blood of an unconscious child can pivot the story toward suspicions of foul play. On the other hand, teens and adults tend to take multiple drugs at once, like chasing oxycodone tablets down with tequila shots or using ecstasy and ketamine together (known as kitty flipping).

FORENSICS

Authors writing scenes involving murder investigations and medical examiners should research specific information about drug detection in blood, urine, tissues, and hair samples after death. Autopsy drug data can be altered by a host of factors, including:

- Which drug was involved
- How much drug was taken

- How the drug was taken (inhaled, injected, swallowed, etc.)
- How long the drug was in the body before death
- The body temperature
- The amount of food in the victim's stomach (for swallowed drugs)
- The length of time since death
- Redistribution and continued metabolism of the drug after death

These details are complex and beyond the scope of this book, but toxicology websites, emergency room physicians, medical examiners, poison centers, and social media groups specializing in forensics and postmortem analysis can be great resources.

ADDITIONAL RESOURCES

Beta readers and critique partners with healthcare backgrounds

Medically knowledgeable beta readers can assess your scenes and dialogue for credibility. They'll know if your emergency room doctor sounds real, if a nurse would behave as you depict, or if emergency medical responders are allowed to give a specific drug.

Include at least one healthcare professional (doctor, nurse, pharmacist, paramedic, etc.) to verify the believability of your scene and dialogue.

Research

There's a wealth of drug information available. A few resources to consider include:

- FDA (Food and Drug Administration) and DEA online databases and drug resources, which provide information on changing trends in various geographic locations as well as updates on the legal status of various drugs.
- Social networking groups focusing on related specialty writing topics, such as trauma or emergency medicine, can be a wealth of information.
- Newspaper articles and medical journals are great places to find real cases.
- Local medical professionals, police, and medical examiners can provide insight and realistic ideas.
- The US national poison center (Poisonhelp.org) is an often-forgotten resource that collects data from fifty-five poison centers throughout the US. It provides free information to the public on poisonings, drug exposure, chemicals, poisonous plants, and

venoms. It's a wealth of information on trends in drug abuse, overdoses, and poisonings based on age groups and geographic locations. The poison center is also available to guide the general public during poisoning emergencies, such as the frantic parents of a toddler found chewing on iron tablets next to an empty vial. The poison center can guide these distraught parents to a local emergency room. They may calculate the toxicity level expected from the iron overdose and even notify the emergency room doctors of the situation.

A Note of Caution: Using Brand Names

An abundance of caution should be used when deciding to use the brand name of a drug in your story. Brand names can be acceptable, but using language that tarnishes, defames, or falsely depicts a product as dangerous can bring litigation. Authors can circumvent these concerns by avoiding the use of brand names entirely. It's often not even necessary to specifically mention a drug name to develop a scene. Use your writing skills to describe how the drug looks, tastes, or makes the character feel, and let the reader fill in pertinent details. Instead of mentioning the brand OxyContin, build tension as the character opens the leftover bottle of pain pills. Instead of Adderall, a stressed college student studying for finals can reach for his "study buddies" bought in a previous scene. Simply describing what the medicine does can be effective, evoking the reader's memory of similar experiences. If you want to be completely fictional, invent your own brand name, but try to stay within the symptoms expected from that kind of drug. Suzanne Collins blended several of these concepts well in *The Hunger Games* series. The sweet syrup that calmed Gale's pain and was extremely addictive was reminiscent of morphine. If you do choose to use a real brand name, consider getting a legal consult to verify that you haven't crossed the boundaries of acceptable use.

Dying to Get to the Fun Stuff?

Chapter 2: Using Toxidromes to Plot That Twist will help you pick out a drug and plausible symptoms to start building your scene. Already have a specific drug or symptoms in mind? The alphabetical index will guide you to chapters with related information to help you develop a compelling scene.

2

USING TOXIDROMES TO PLOT THAT TWIST

How can an emergency room (ER) doctor treat an unconscious overdose patient without knowing which drug was taken? Doctors can't instantly measure drug levels, and there are no miracle antidotes that work in every situation. ER doctors often act like medical detectives, matching a patient's symptoms with possible causes. When doctors suspect a drug overdose or poisoning, they can use toxidromes to piece the puzzle together.

For doctors, toxidromes help match a group of symptoms with a list of suspected causes. For authors, toxidromes provide plausible drug-symptom combinations for plotting drug scenes.

SETTING THE SCENE

To apply a toxidrome to a scene, consider these questions:

Which drug should be in the scene?

> *Not sure which drug to pick?* Look over the toxidrome drug-symptom tables for a combination fitting your concept.

> *Have you already picked a drug?* Find a list of possible symptoms for the drug using the tables. Does the drug still fit your proposed scene? Some drugs, such as kratom or inhalants, may not fit nicely into a specific toxidrome. If your drug isn't listed in a toxidrome, check the table of contents for a related chapter. Still can't find your drug? Use the index of symptoms to pick another drug that offers similar risks for your scene.

Which (and how many) symptoms should you use?

> *Non-overdose scene.* Choose one to two less serious symptoms to add depth to a character's behavior. Adding a few more symptoms is reasonable as long as it doesn't start to sound like a checklist.

Overdose scene. The character should also develop several of the more serious symptoms.

How should the scene develop?

Once you've picked the best drug-symptom combination for your scenario, refer to the individual drug chapter for suggestions on developing a believable progression of those symptoms, including how the character will act or feel, how quickly symptoms should start, how much peril to place the character in, and how to spin a page-turner. Sample scenarios and writing prompts are included to get your creativity flowing.

Let's dive in!

Table 2.1 The Opioid Toxidrome

If the Scene Includes	
Codeine	Meperidine (Demerol)*
Dextromethorphan (see	Methadone
Hallucinogen Toxidrome)	Morphine
Fentanyl	Opium
Heroin	Oxycodone (OxyContin, Percocet, Percodan)
Hydrocodone*	Tramadol (Ultram)*
Hydromorphone (Dilaudid)	

Possible Character Symptoms Include*		
Lower Dose:	Higher Dose *(previous symptoms plus)*:	Dangerously High Dose *(previous symptoms plus)*:
• Slowed thinking • Drowsiness	• Euphoria ("high," a floating sense of well-being) • Slurred speech • Nausea, vomiting • Poor coordination (clumsy, staggering, fumbling) • Pinpoint pupils (reserve this symptom for a medical character to identify) • Disorientation • Confusion	• Severe confusion • Slowed breathing (or stopped completely) • Cold clammy skin, blue lips, and/or blue nail beds • Slowed heart rate • Seizures (especially with meperidine) • Loss of consciousness • Coma

Not specifically described in chapter 13. Symptoms for tramadol and hydrocodone will be similar to those of oxycodone; meperidine symptoms are similar to those of morphine with the added risk of seizures; symptoms listed may overlap between columns.

Table 2.2 Sedative-Hypnotic Toxidrome

If the Scene Includes

Alcohol	Chloral Hydrate
"Anxiety pills"	GHB
Barbiturates, including:	"Sleeping pills"
• Phenobarbital	
• Sodium Thiopental	

"Benzos" (benzodiazepines), including*:
• Alprazolam (Xanax)
• Diazepam (Valium)*
• Flunitrazepam (Rohypnol, Roofies)
• Lorazepam (Ativan)*
• Midazolam (Versed)

Possible Character Symptoms Include

Lower Dose	Higher Dose *(previous symptoms plus)*:
• Drowsiness	• Sedation
• Slightly poor coordination (clumsy)	• Confusion (significant)
• Slurred speech	• Very poor coordination (staggering, fumbling, walking into objects)
	• Difficulty thinking/foggy brain
	• Slowed breathing
	• Slowed heart rate
	• Decreased blood pressure
	• Hallucinations
	• Delirium
	• Coma

Tips:
"Benzos" may not decrease breathing unless taken in very high doses or combined with other drugs/alcohol. Barbiturates can cause dangerously slowed (or stopped) breathing. Other: Amnesia with benzodiazepines

Lorazepam and diazepam are not specifically discussed in the benzodiazepine section, but in general can cause your character symptoms similar to those of alprazolam.

Table 2.3 Stimulant Toxidrome

If the Scene Includes

Amphetamines: • Methamphetamine (Meth) • Prescription stimulants: Methylphenidate (Ritalin), Amphetamine/dextroamphetamine (Adderall)	Bath Salts Caffeine Cocaine Ecstasy (Molly, MDMA, see Hallucinogen Toxidrome) Pseudoephedrine Spice/K2 (*see* Hallucinogen Toxidrome)

Possible Character Symptoms Include

Lower doses • Hyperactivity (high energy levels, animation, speaking a lot or fast) • Hyperalert • Insomnia • Decreased hunger	Higher doses *(previous symptoms plus)*: • Tremors (such as hands shaking) • Sweating a LOT • Extreme agitation • Severe headache • Blunted feeling of pain (specifically cocaine, bath salts, meth) • Fast heart rate • High blood pressure • High body temperature • Seizures • Chest pain • Heart attack • Stroke Also with meth: Jaws and/or fists tightly clenched, paranoia (perceived threats)

Table 2.4 Anticholinergic Toxidrome*

If the Scene Includes

Antihistamines (diphenhydramine, nonprescription insomnia or allergy medicines)
Antidepressants (*mostly* older "tricyclic antidepressants")
Atropine
Belladonna
Jimson weed
Scopolamine

Possible Character Symptoms Include

Lower doses:	High doses (*previous symptoms plus*):
• Dry mouth	• Very dry mouth ("cotton mouth")
• Sedation, tiredness	• Flushed/hot/dry skin
	• Decreased sweating
	• Increased body temperature
	• Inability to focus on a conversation
	• Agitation
	• Hallucinations
	• Delirium
	• Full bladder, but can't urinate
	• Fast heart rate
	• Very dilated eyes (enlarged pupils; reserve for a medical character to identify)
	• Seizures

* *There's a mnemonic in medicine used to describe the typical overdose symptoms with these drugs:*
Blind as a bat (blurry vision, dilated pupils)
Red as a beet (flushed red skin)
Dry as a bone (dry mouth)
Full as a flask (can't urinate, full bladder)
Hot as a hare (increased body temperature)
and
Mad as a hatter (agitation, hallucinations, delirium, seizures)

Table 2.5 Hallucinogen Toxidrome

If the Scene Includes	
Dextromethorphan (DXM, see Opioid Toxidrome)	Magic Mushrooms
	Marijuana
Ecstasy (Molly, MDMA)	Mescaline/Peyote
Ketamine	Spice/K2 (see Stimulant Toxidrome)
LSD (acid)	

Possible Character Symptoms Include

- Confusion
- Disorientation
- Agitation
- Fast heart rate
- Fast breathing rate
- High blood pressure
- Hallucinations
- Delusions
- Psychotic behavior
- Coma

3

A WORD ABOUT ANTIDOTES

Despite what you may have seen in movies, there are few antidotes for drug overdoses. Most of the time, doctors must rely on supportive care, such as giving oxygen, intravenous fluids, and medications to control severe symptoms, such as seizures, until the patient improves. The approach used is different depending on the potential drug involved and the recommendations for treatment periodically change based on new research. For example, syrup of ipecac was a household staple in the 1960s. It was used to cause vomiting for certain kinds of overdoses and poisonings. Over time, as research proved the risks of ipecac outweighed the benefits, it was removed from emergency treatment guidelines and, eventually, the US market by the early 2000s. Even those "pumping the stomach" scenes may not be appropriate. This process, known as gastric lavage, isn't done as often anymore—it doesn't work in many situations and can cause more harm than other treatments.

However, for some drug overdoses, there are antidotes that can realistically be used in scenes. These include naloxone (Narcan), widely known as a potential lifesaver in opioid overdoses, and flumazenil (Romazicon), which can be used for benzodiazepine overdoses.

Having an overdosed character's stomach pumped will be dramatic, but often wrong.

A few tips for using these rescue drugs in scenes are included below. Since these scenes can become very complicated, avoid the temptation of detailing each step of the antidote rescue. Painting the general picture for the reader will be effective and avoid a flawed description. Picking the right antidote will be important for believability. Then, as you weave the scene, let your reader worry about the antidote working and the character surviving, not the exact details of how it's given. Also, consult a medical professional to ensure the scene seems plausible. This is especially true if your overdose plot does not fit the scenarios detailed below.

Naloxone (Narcan)

Only use this antidote in opioid overdose scenes. Naloxone won't work to reverse most other drugs. It can be used in scenes involving fentanyl, heroin, or oxycodone, for example, but not methamphetamine or cocaine (unless it's suspected that these drugs were contaminated with fentanyl or your character was taking multiple drugs). However, it's not wrong for naloxone to be given to an unconscious overdosed character that isn't breathing—even if no one is sure what drug was taken. At best, it will help; at worst, it won't hurt.

Research your timeline. Opioid overdoses have been rapidly increasing since the early 1990s due in part to an oversupply of opioid pain pills from overprescribing. With the declaration of an opioid crisis in 2017, opioid prescribing restrictions were enacted. But when prescription sources of oxycodone dried up, some users turned to street oxycodone, resulting in ongoing opioid deaths. As street oxycodone and many other drugs began to be laced by drug traffickers with deadly amounts of fentanyl, another wave of overdoses began and continues today. If your scene occurs before the opioid crisis, naloxone would have mostly been available in medical settings (hospitals, doctors' offices, or via emergency medical responders). Since 2017 most states have passed legislation to expand naloxone access to the general public by allowing pharmacists to dispense it without a prescription and requiring them to provide training and information about its proper use. The public has been encouraged to buy naloxone to keep on hand, in case of an emergency. So, while your character in 2020 can't just go into any store and buy naloxone off the shelf, he can buy it from a pharmacist in many states. In some areas of the US, cities provide the public with vending machines stocked with free naloxone and organizations hand out free antidote kits to homeless encampments, where overdoses have been escalating. In 2023, the Food and Drug Administration (FDA) approved naloxone to be sold over the counter throughout the US. So, soon your character *will* be able to buy it in almost any store.

Over the last few years, wider access to naloxone has helped save countless people from overdose deaths. However, the increased demand for naloxone has depleted supplies in some areas, making the antidote unavailable, offering a believable complication for a scene.

Become familiar with how naloxone is given. In hospitals, your scene will generally involve either injecting the antidote or using a nose spray. In some cases, the doctor or nurse uses a syringe that's been prepackaged with the correct dose. In other cases, the antidote must be measured out of a vial into a syringe during the emergency, creating a stressful, error-prone situation. This dose, then, is either injected into a vein or, with a special syringe adaptor, sprayed into the nose. Thankfully, the general public has access to simpler products: an automatic syringe injector and a nose spray. Most recently, a high dose of naloxone has been developed to combat overdoses from increasingly potent street opioids. Pictures of these various products can be found online using keywords such as *naloxone, naloxone syringes, naloxone nasal,* or *naloxone instructions.* Online training videos are available for the naloxone nose spray and the automatic injector. Watching these videos makes it easier to understand how to depict a character using them. Want an in-person demonstration? Ask a local pharmacist to teach you how to give the naloxone nose spray using one of their training kits.

Ask for a demonstration of a naloxone antidote device at your local pharmacy.

No instant effects. Your character should not suddenly start breathing, talking, and walking after a naloxone dose. In real life, it can take about two to five minutes for naloxone to begin working, and rescue breathing is sometimes needed in the meantime to avoid brain damage or death. Your overdosed character has probably passed out and his breathing is getting very slow or has stopped completely. His lips and fingertips may be turning blueish. After naloxone is given, a believable scene would include this character starting to slowly breathe over the next few minutes, his mind sluggish and foggy. As his breathing improves, the blue tinge to his lips should begin fading back to pink. Several more minutes should pass before he begins thinking a little more clearly, even longer to feel strong enough to sit or stand. But if you're writing a naloxone rescue scene for an unconscious character with an opioid addiction, it's plausible for him to wake up much more rapidly, yelling, agitated, thrashing, hitting people within reach, and angry his high was ruined. The naloxone will also cause him to be in immediate opioid withdrawal.

Unfortunately, if your character was taking the opioid for severe pain, naloxone will reverse *all* of the drug's effects and the pain will quickly return.

When you don't want everything to work out. Sometimes, you just want to add another twist to keep your readers on the edge. There are several complications that can occur with naloxone to consider.

- *The antidote doesn't work.* Maybe your character didn't actually overdose on an opioid, but something else. The naloxone won't work and the scene can spiral into a page-turner, with your character still in peril. Or did your character accidentally overdose on fentanyl-tainted marijuana? Many street drugs have increasingly contained dangerous amounts of fentanyl and fentanyl cousins that are so potent that more than one rescue dose is needed to restart a victim's breathing. Sometimes, the naloxone hasn't worked at all. This may be because another drug was also involved or the victim already had irreversible brain damage from a lack of oxygen.
- *The antidote wears off too soon.* Naloxone is a temporary remedy—after several minutes, its effects wear off. When the overdose has been caused by a long-acting drug (such as extended release tablets), after the naloxone wears off, overdose symptoms can reoccur, leaving rescuers scrambling to find another dose of antidote and keeping your readers on the edge of their seats.
- *Seizures.* Is your character addicted to opioids? If he overdoses, a rescue dose of naloxone will not only help him breathe but also send him into rapid withdrawal, potentially inducing seizures. Your character's entire body may be convulsing, causing drool or foam to drip from his mouth.

If you're looking for a nefarious angle to this twist, consider an unscrupulous detective using naloxone to trigger rapid opioid withdrawal in a suspect to get information. When the suspect refuses to divulge his secrets, the detective may let him suffer before giving him a hit of heroin to ease the symptoms. *Now,* will the threat of more naloxone be enough to get the suspect to confess all he knows? Or maybe the detective threatens to give him a heroin overdose.

Flumazenil (Romazicon)

Only use this antidote in benzodiazepine overdose scenes. It won't work for most other types of drug overdoses.

Research your timeline. While flumazenil was accidentally discovered decades ago, it wasn't approved for use in the US until 2004. Prior to then, there wasn't a benzodiazepine antidote.

Become familiar with how it's given. Flumazenil is only available as an injection and in a medical setting. Ask medical personnel for information on how it's used in emergencies. This is not an antidote available to the general public, so your character shouldn't have doses stored at his home or buy it at a local pharmacy.

No instant effects. Your character should not suddenly start breathing, talking, and walking after a flumazenil dose. Similar to naloxone in opioid toxicity, your character should remain mentally groggy for some time after the antidote is given. Have him take several minutes to think more clearly and even longer before trying to get up.

When you don't want everything to work out. If you want to add another twist to keep your readers on the edge, there's a complication with flumazenil to consider.

- *Seizures.* Flumazenil can trigger withdrawal, including seizures, in chronic benzodiazepine abusers. To make it more complicated, benzodiazepines also happen to be one of the fastest ways to stop a seizure. With that flumazenil dose, your protagonist has not only caused seizures in that poor character but also made him resistant to the very drug that could stop them.

PUTTING IT ALL TOGETHER

Sample Scenario Kam finds his friend Jesse unconscious on the bathroom floor next to an empty syringe. He shakes Jesse, yells his name, but nothing happens. Jesse's lips are blue, his breathing barely noticeable. Kam fumbles in the drawer for the naloxone and quickly squirts a dose up Jesse's nose. He waits, watching, his eyes brimming with tears. Finally, Jesse's chest starts rising and falling, the blue tinge to his lips slowly fading.

Now you try it

Writing Prompt Rewrite the scene above. What happens when Jesse gets the naloxone if he's addicted to opioids? Does he wake slowly? Or does he wake in a rage? How does this scene end?

4

ALCOHOL

Brief History/Social Context

The rich history of alcohol use in society and its impact on people will offer a wide range of ways to enrich your story and characters. References to alcohol can be casually woven into scenes, such as an older couple sipping champagne at an elegant party or a wounded Civil War soldier chugging a bottle of whiskey before an amputation. It can form the focus of a scene—the beer pong game at a high school party. Or your character's life may be changed by alcohol—the poor farmer selling moonshine to make a living during Prohibition or the child of an abusive drunk parent.

Regardless, due to the vast changes over time in social acceptance, trends, and laws, research will be a key aspect to believability. For example, you don't want to make the mistake of having your protagonist buy wine on Christmas morning in Oklahoma City in the 1970s, where restrictive laws kept liquor stores closed on holidays.

The extensive array of alcohols and their uses is far beyond the scope of this book. Instead, this chapter will focus on how alcohol can affect your character and a few of its unusual or trendy uses (and the related dangers) to consider for your story.

Rubbing alcohol

Rubbing alcohol is best known for its use to ward off infection from cuts and punctures (like vaccines). But there are several dangerous uses of rubbing alcohol that may offer creative options for writers.

Rubbing alcohol baths. Rubbing alcohol baths have been used for generations as a folk remedy to reduce fevers, especially in children. The feverish person may soak in bathwater mixed with rubbing alcohol, have an alcohol-soaked sponge bath, or even wrap an alcohol-saturated towel around their head. Your story twist? Alcohol baths not only don't work but they can be lethal, especially in children.

Why do people believe this method works? Because rubbing alcohol evaporates so rapidly that it chills the person's skin, causing them to shiver and making them look cooler. But shivering actually *raises* body temperature. Shivering is a natural physical response to cold—it's the body trying to warm itself by making the muscles generate heat. So while a character's mom is happy that her son's *skin* is cooling down, she won't realize his *internal* temperature is increasing. It could even climb fast enough to cause seizures. To make matters worse, inhaling the alcohol vapors can cause the character to suffer alcohol poisoning, with severe mental confusion, strained breathing, and vomiting. He could lapse into a coma and even die. Despite the risks and a number of reported deaths since the 1950s, rubbing alcohol baths are still practiced in some families today.

Don't have a rubbing alcohol bath cure your character's high fever.

Drinking rubbing alcohol. Drinking rubbing alcohol can be lethal. Rubbing alcohol is a mixture of isopropyl alcohol, water, and often other ingredients, such as oil of wintergreen. It's widely available and cheap, which unfortunately makes it tempting for some poor alcoholics to drink. And drinking just a few ounces of rubbing alcohol can be lethal. Your character will seem drunk. He'll be dizzy, his stomach will hurt, and he might vomit blood. When his breathing becomes dangerously slow he'll pass out. Without emergency medical help, he can slip into a coma and die. In small children, drinking rubbing alcohol is even more dangerous, with as little as a teaspoon causing lethal alcohol intoxication.

Your penniless alcoholic character can become rapidly toxic from drinking cheap rubbing alcohol and even die.

Calorie avoidance/breathalyzer tests

Calorie avoidance myths have spurred attempts by "slimmers" and some models to avoid alcohol calories by either inserting an alcohol-soaked tampon (which makes the vagina or rectum burn) or by snorting alcohol (making the nose tissue burn). These same approaches have been tried by teens

Don't have a character pass a breathalyzer test after getting drunk—no matter how the alcohol was consumed.

attempting to get drunk with less alcohol and avoid failing breathalyzer tests. But if your protagonist tries either of these methods, they won't work for any of these goals. It's unlikely that your character will get drunk after a single alcohol-soaked tampon or snorting alcohol. Even a saturated super-sized tampon can only hold one to two shots of alcohol and would be very difficult to use, with much of the alcohol leaking out as it's inserted. As an added disincentive, the alcohol can cause painful, irritated skin, leaving your character miserable. And snorting enough alcohol to get drunk would require a lot of volume that could leave your character sputtering as the liquid burns her nasal tissue and drips down her throat. If she does manage to consume enough alcohol to get a buzz, not only will she have consumed calories, but the alcohol will register on a breathalyzer.

Alcohol enemas

Alcohol enemas are for the rowdy college party scene that ends very badly. This dangerous practice goes by various names, including *boofing, butt chugging,* or *butt beer bong.* The alcohol is poured through a tube that has been inserted into the "drinker's" rectum. *Why* would anyone do this? The goal is to get drunk faster with less alcohol. And it works . . . it's just also potentially lethal. Alcohol absorbs rapidly as an enema and there's no way to stop the process. If a small amount of alcohol is used, your character can become buzzed. But if a large amount is used, any alcohol that's already in the intestines will keep absorbing, even after your character's dangerously drunk. And while her body might try to force some of the alcohol out, using an enema bypasses the body's major safety mechanism to avoid lethal intoxication—vomiting. Ultimately, the enema can lead to alcohol poisoning and death.

A party scene involving alcohol enemas can believably end in death from alcohol poisoning.

Alcohol inhalation (vaping alcohol)

Alcohol inhalation is a process that involves creating alcohol vapors to inhale, either by heating it or dropping it onto dry ice. Special devices have even been marketed to create these vapors. As the alcohol is inhaled, it passes quickly through the lungs and into the brain. Inhaled alcohol is much more intoxicating than drinking the same volume. If your character isn't careful, he won't realize how drunk he's getting and will keep inhaling the vapors. This can quickly turn from a character that's slightly drunk to one that's on the brink of death from alcohol poisoning.

Jell-O shots

Jell-O shots are made with alcohol-infused gelatin and are quite trendy in a wide range of ages, from youth to adults. You can just as easily pen these into a party scene involving high school students as one involving retirees. The alcoholic mixture is often served in small cups or prefilled syringes. What makes Jell-O shots so popular? The gelatin flavor masks the presence of alcohol, and the colorful, bouncy gelatin is reminiscent of a childhood treat, making these "edible alcohols" seem fun and more acceptable. Despite these being trendy, the concept of thickening alcohol with some form of flavored gelatin can be found in recipe books dating back several generations. The recipes vary by the amount and kind of alcohol used, but tequila, vodka, and rum are typical. And while many people still make their own gelatin shots, premade shots are available to buy in bulk for parties.

So, just how many gelatin shots *does* your character need to slurp up before realistically becoming drunk? There's no specific answer, due to the wide variety of alcohol content in the shots. Some shots contain very little, while others contain so much alcohol that they're more like a thickened liquid. Some are single shots, while some are made double-sized. At the very least, with the most concentrated recipe, your character should be prepared to swallow somewhere between three to four regular sized shots to equal about the same amount of alcohol as one standard shot of liquor (less if it was made using concentrated grain alcohol—which is illegal in some states). That can be a *lot* of sugary Jell-O to drink before feeling a buzz.

Don't have a character get drunk after just a couple of Jell-O shots.

Methanol/Wood alcohol

Methanol is a common impurity found in moonshine, hooch, or any other name that can be given to home-distilled liquor. Remember that farmer I mentioned at the beginning of this chapter, the one selling moonshine? If he's drinking the moonshine he made, and it contains methanol, he's in a lot of danger. The problem? Methanol is metabolized in the liver to extremely toxic chemicals that cause blindness, seizures, coma, and death. In an adult, just a *couple of ounces* is lethal; in a child, a small mouthful can be deadly.

Frighteningly, during the COVID-19 pandemic, some hand sanitizing gels were marketed that contained methanol, instead of the typical isopropyl alcohol. And since methanol can rapidly absorb across the skin, several deaths occurred.

Still looking for ideas?

There are an endless number of creative ways people attempt intoxication. But don't be tempted to write a scene based on social media trends. Some of the wilder methods bragged about on social media may not actually work. Worse, they can be dangerous or lethal if actually tried. For example, one trend involved pouring alcohol onto your eyeball in an attempt to get drunk. Not only was it painful and damaging to the eye but so little alcohol was absorbed that it didn't even cause intoxication. Curious authors interested in more information on these and other unique scene options involving alcohol can search online using keywords like *eyeballing, smoking alcohol, vaping alcohol, snorting alcohol,* and *get drunk without drinking.*

Slang Terms

(There are a wide variety of terms for alcohol, but the list here will specifically refer to the unusual uses of alcohol described in this chapter.)

Street names

- For moonshine: dew, firewater, hooch, moonshine, mountain dew, white lightening
- For alcohol enemas: butt bong, stinky drinky, up-the-hatch
- For Jell-O shots: jellies, shots

Other terms

- Butt chugging, boofing: alcohol inserted into the rectum.
- Slimmers: people who ingest alcohol without drinking (for example, alcohol-soaked tampons), mistakenly believing that the calories are reduced or absent.
- Vaptini: inhaling/vaping alcohol fumes.

Weaving the Plot

How is it used?

Rubbing alcohol is wiped on the skin to cleanse it and reduce infection from cuts, scrapes, or injections. To make baths, rubbing alcohol is poured into the water in either a bathtub or a bowl (for a sponge bath). When alcohol tampons are used, the tampons are soaked in alcohol, then inserted into either the vagina or the rectum. To inhale alcohol, it can be poured over dry ice, boiled on the stove, put into various containers to heat the liquor, or sometimes added to an asthma nebulizer. For enemas, the alcohol is poured into a funnel attached to a tube placed into the rectum. The funnel is usually hung higher than the body so the alcohol will drain into the body. Methanol should *not* be purposefully used, as it's extremely toxic. However, it can be accidentally ingested, such as by a character who buys moonshine. Methanol-containing hand sanitizers were briefly marketed during the COVID-19 pandemic but were removed from the market due to severe illness and deaths.

Now you try it

> **Writing Prompt #1** Develop a scene where your character believes in old-fashioned rubbing alcohol baths and plans to use one for a feverish child. (You'll continue this scene in Writing Prompt #2.)

How will my character act or feel?

For scenes that involve your main character getting drunk, the progression of symptoms can go from feeling a mild buzz to staggering and slurring words to the extreme of a blackout, coma, and death. If the character has had a few Jell-O shots, your character may simply become relaxed, more sociable, and feel giddy. But if she drinks enough of them, she can be drowsy, clumsy, slur her speech, and have difficulty thinking.

Want a drunk character to not remember the party later? It's plausible. With alcohol, a "blackout" can happen where the events that take place while drunk are completely forgotten despite the person seeming to be awake at the time.

Other serious dangers for your very drunk character include seizures, choking on vomit, very slow (or stopped) breathing, a coma, or death. If you're curious about symptoms associated with specific blood alcohol levels, an online calculator with a table of related symptoms can be found using the search phrase *blood alcohol content calculator.*

A blackout can keep your character from remembering the awful thing she did while drunk.

Alcohol can alter your character's personality. It can cause a wide spectrum of behaviors, from a chatty, happy partier to an angry, abusive drunk. And depending on the character, these behaviors can happen after just a little or a lot of alcohol.

In addition to the typical alcohol side effects, there are some symptoms associated specifically with the unique methods of using alcohol discussed in this chapter. Drinking rubbing alcohol will cause your character to rapidly become drunk, with a severe headache, dizziness, stomach pain, nausea, and possibly bloody vomit. Her breath will smell sweet, like nail polish remover. After drinking only a few ounces, she can also pass out, have slow, labored breathing, and possibly die.

For scenes including rubbing alcohol baths, the alcohol will evaporate from your character's skin rapidly, making her shiver and raising her core body temperature. The increasing effects from the vapors, such as mental confusion, a bad headache, or vomiting, can even be mistaken as more signs of whatever illness caused the fever. With enough vapors, when your character gets out of the tub, she'll be dizzy, confused, and stumbling. Her heart will be pounding. When she collapses to the floor, unconscious, her breathing will sound painfully strained and she could die without emergency help.

Vaping the equivalent of a single alcoholic drink will cause a drunkenness similar to swallowing a couple of drinks, but much more rapidly. The initial alcohol buzz might temporarily pass, making your character assume she hasn't inhaled enough to get drunk, so she'll inhale more. When the second wave of symptoms hits, she'll suddenly feel extremely drunk. She'll stumble, fall, slur words, and not be able to think clearly. You can decide the level of peril for this character. She can pass out, be barely breathing, lapse into a coma, and even die.

Alcohol tampons will cause tissue burning that can last for several hours or longer, leaving your poor character in pain.

Alcohol enemas can be rapidly lethal for a character.

An alcohol enema will cause your character's rectal tissue to have a burning sensation as soon as any alcohol touches her skin. If the pain makes her stop the enema now, she can be fine or even slightly drunk. If she keeps pouring more alcohol into her body, she'll start slurring her words within just a few minutes and rapidly progress to drowsy and confused. Then, there will be nothing that she can do to stop the rest of that alcohol already in her intestines from absorbing. Does she realize her grave situation as she passes out? This scene will end badly for this character.

With methanol poisoning, over the first few hours, your character will rapidly become confused, get a severe headache, have blurry vision, become nauseated, and feel dizzy. That farmer drinking his own moonshine may think that he's just drunk, but soon he'll be vomiting, staggering, and very confused. His heart will be racing and he may have trouble breathing. Eventually, he'll collapse, seizing. Coma and death will rapidly follow. If he gets emergency medical help, he could survive but he might be blind.

Now you try it

> **Writing Prompt #2** Continue your scene from Writing Prompt #1. Partway through the child's bath, the mom begins to realize something is wrong with how her child is acting. Does she figure out the problem before her child is deathly ill?

How long will this drug affect my character?

Many variables impact how long the effects of alcohol last, including the number of drinks, how large the character is, and how recently food was eaten. In general, the initial effects from an alcoholic drink (like light-headedness and relaxation) will start within ten to fifteen minutes. The full effects can take another ten to fifteen minutes to develop. So, if the character quickly drank several shots of alcohol, in about thirty minutes she'll realize *just* how drunk she is. Symptoms from vaping alcohol can begin within a few seconds to a minute since the alcohol vapor is so concentrated and goes quickly to the brain. With alcohol baths it can take several minutes (ten to fifteen) to inhale enough fumes to feel the symptoms beginning. Alcohol tampons won't cause your character to get drunk, but skin-burning sensations can start within seconds. Even after the tampon is removed, the character's skin can be very irritated and remain extremely tender for several more hours or longer. Symptoms from alcohol enemas can appear within a few minutes (less than five) and continue to worsen as long as the alcohol in the intestines keeps absorbing.

Once alcohol is in a person's body, the effects can last for several hours. Some references say it takes at least an hour for a body to remove the equivalent of a single drink, although breathalyzer tests can still be positive for alcohol the following day. Online graphs can show how long your character may reasonably seem drunk depending upon the amount of alcohol consumed. It's important to note that *nothing* can speed up the process of becoming sober—not caffeine, not fluids, not food. After all, the liver can only clear alcohol so fast, no matter what. Instead of an espresso suddenly making a drunk character sober, a more honest scene would have that caffeine create a

It's not realistic to depict a drunk character as suddenly sober after drinking coffee.

more alert drunk that believes she's fine, without realizing how impaired she remains. She might think she can drive herself home, but that could be a deadly mistake.

It's very hard to determine how long the effects may last from alcohol *fumes*. For vaping, a reasonable approach is to depict the character's intoxication as similar to consuming several times the amount of alcohol she vaped. Did she vape about two shots of alcohol? She should act like she chugged four shots instead. For fumes from alcohol baths, mild symptoms can begin decreasing within a few minutes of being away from the source. A headache, for example, can recede over about thirty minutes to an hour. However, if your character was very dizzy, nauseous, vomiting, and passing out, it's time to have your readers worry about medical help arriving before she ends up in a coma or dies.

PUTTING IT ALL TOGETHER

Sample Scenario She slammed back another vodka, forcing herself not to puke and pushed back from the bar, knocking over a chair. Giggling, she gripped the edge of the bar as she swayed. She felt a hand on her shoulder.

"I'll go with you."

"I can go by myself," she snapped, pushing Nia's hand away, then stumbled toward the bathroom.

Now you try it

Writing Prompt #3 Write a scene involving a group of women that are drinking Jell-O shots at a retirement party. How do they act? Who made the shots. What's the party like? Have some fun with this one!

5

ANTIDEPRESSANTS

Brief History/Social Context

Several generations of antidepressants have been developed since they were first used in the 1950s. The oldest, called "tricyclic antidepressants" (TCAs), such as amitriptyline, have a long history of being used for intentional overdoses. With the advent of newer antidepressants in the mid-1980s, such as the SSRIs (selective serotonin reuptake inhibitors), TCAs have become much less prescribed for depression. They're still used in a few chronic pain conditions, however. These newer antidepressants are considered safer, although in extremely high doses or combined with alcohol, they can still be lethal. So, while your attempted overdose scene set in the 1970s could involve a TCA, one set in 2020 could include either a TCA or one of the newer antidepressants. Despite decreased prescribing, TCAs remain responsible for the highest percentage of overdose deaths from antidepressants, usually involving more women than men.

With a TCA overdose, your character should develop several symptoms from the Anticholinergic Toxidrome, such as severe confusion, seizures, a coma, or even death. With an SSRI overdose, she can believably survive, suffering drowsiness, nausea, and vomiting. But for more dramatic symptoms, the SSRI can cause the potentially lethal Serotonin Syndrome (see "How will my character act or feel?" below). Or if the character is drinking alcohol with the SSRI, her condition can deteriorate to include seizures, coma, and death.

Your character can believably survive an SSRI overdose.

There are a few important points to consider when choosing to plot an overdose scene with an antidepressant. With the complexity of the different kinds of antidepressants, each with different overdose risks and symptoms, the simplest approach is to avoid specifics, such as naming the drug. Instead, let the reader add their own details as the scene unfolds: a distraught, depressed teen, her face red, streaked with tears, opening her mom's prescription bottle, pouring the contents into her hand. This character should develop some overdose symptoms common to a variety of antidepressants, such as drowsiness, confusion, seizures, and a loss of consciousness. This avoids depicting a wrong drug-symptom combination yet still allows you to build tension.

Slang Terms

(Since terminology and slang terms change over time, further research is highly encouraged.)

Street names

blue angels, blue birds, happy pills, TCAs

Weaving the Plot

How is it used?

Antidepressants are usually capsules or pills.

Now you try it

> **Writing Prompt #1** Develop the background for a character who's considering an overdose of antidepressants. What led to this emotionally charged moment? Where will the character get the pills? (You'll use this information in Writing Prompt #2.)

How will my character act or feel?

The first hour after a high dose of a TCA, your character can begin to enjoy a sociable high. But she can also feel drowsy, with a dry mouth and blurry vision. She can continue to feel worse, becoming shaky, with a rapid heartbeat and a headache. Large amounts of pills can lead to nausea, causing her to vomit. If she vomits enough of the pills or didn't take enough to die, her symptoms *might* resolve on their own over the next day or two.

But, if she took a potentially lethal dose, by about two hours after taking the pills, your character will be in great peril, suffering a pounding heartbeat, dizziness, and confusion. She may see, hear, or talk to people that aren't there and behave erratically. For example, your character could realistically have a conversation with a wall or search in the backyard for the butter for her toast. She can suffer a brief seizure that may leave her unconscious, or have several seizures that continue nonstop. If they continue, if you're not planning to have emergency medical help arrive during the scene, the character should not survive. Even with medical help, her heart and blood pressure may not respond to the emergency drugs and she could suffer a heart attack.

Hallucinations are possible with TCA overdoses.

With newer antidepressants, like the SSRIs, your overdosing character can suffer nausea, vomiting, drowsiness, and a rapid, pounding heartbeat. If a night of drinking is mixed with all those SSRI pills, coma and/or death can believably end the scene. Even without any alcohol, high SSRIs doses can also cause Serotonin Syndrome, which can cause your character to sweat, shiver, have a tremor (shakes), and a rapid heartbeat. In a severe case, Serotonin Syndrome can be lethal. Your character will become agitated, confused, and have a severe headache. She could then suffer a seizure, pass out, stop breathing, and die.

Now you try it

> **Writing Prompt #2** Continue the scene from Writing Prompt #1, starting after the character has taken the overdose. How does the character act around others as the symptoms evolve? How does the scene end?

How long will this drug affect my character?

Milder symptoms from a high dose can last for twenty-four to forty-eight hours, such as mental fogginess and sleepiness. With a potentially lethal dose, symptoms can develop slowly over the first hour, becoming life-threatening within two hours. Characters rescued from an overdose can experience a hangover effect, with brain fog, sleepiness, and poor functioning that lasts many days or even a week after the incident. If a lethal dose is being depicted, medical help should arrive within two to three hours for your character to realistically avoid death.

Sample Scenario #1 The faces in the circle of people stare back at me, some distant, some hopeful—all knowing what I did, why I'm here. I can barely even remember that night. The blurry room, the pain as my head hit the floor, Mom's distant scream. Then nothing. Nothing until I woke strapped to a bed, an IV stinging my arm, hushed sounds nearby, beeps from a machine.

They say I was lucky. That I'd been seizing, my head bleeding badly.

I stared at the faces yearning to hear my story, to fix my problems. Or maybe just to hear about someone worse off and feel better about themselves. But they'll never understand. The fact I'm still alive is the worst luck I've ever had.

Sample Scenario #2 Skyler heads toward the laughter in the family room, but stumbles, grabbing onto the railing, dropping her empty pill bottle. The room swirls slowly, her eyes trying to close.

Now you try it

Writing Prompt #3 Finish the scene with Skyler, above. How does the scene unfold? Does her family find her before it's too late?

6

ANTIHISTAMINES

Brief History/Social Context

Did you know that a simple nonprescription allergy pill can cause your character to hallucinate or even die? Originally developed in the 1940s, antihistamines are used to dry up runny noses, combat allergy symptoms (like itching), quiet coughs, and help with insomnia. They are in cold pills, allergy tablets, and sleep aids.

They can also be lethal.

Just taking a few times more than the typical daily dose can lead to a variety of dangerous symptoms that can include hallucinations, seizures, and death. An interesting way for writers to remember the symptoms your character could suffer from an antihistamine overdose is with a mnemonic used by medical professionals: blind as a bat, red as a beet, dry as a bone, full as a flask, hot as a hare, and mad as a hatter.

Would you be surprised to learn that diphenhydramine, a popularly used nonprescription antihistamine, ranks among the top ten to fifteen drugs used in intentional overdose deaths, not far behind drugs like fentanyl? In fact, before 2020, most diphenhydramine overdoses were associated with attempted suicides. However, in 2020 a widely viewed social media challenge urged viewers to take high diphenhydramine doses to purposefully cause hallucinations. Unfortunately, diphenhydramine doses high enough to cause hallucinations can also be lethal, and

Blind as a bat
(blurry vision, dilated pupils)

Red as a beet
(flushed red skin)

Dry as a bone
(dry mouth)

Full as a flask
(can't urinate, full bladder)

Hot as a hare
(increased body temperature)

Mad as a hatter
(agitation, hallucinations, delirium, seizures)

Common allergy tablets can cause your character to hallucinate . . . or die.

several teens in the US died from participating in the challenge.

There are several generations of antihistamines. The so-called first generation are the older, sedating antihistamines, like diphenhydramine. The newer generations, like loratadine, claim to cause less sedation. While all antihistamines can be dangerous in high doses, the risks differ with various generations and can get quite complicated. But diphenhydramine remains the most popularly abused antihistamine for its ability to cause hallucinations and delirium. Because of this, if you're writing an antihistamine overdose, consider either using diphenhydramine in the scene or simply avoid mentioning the specific drug. Instead, you can let your readers fill in the details, as your character opens a box of allergy medicine, slowly popping each pink pill from the blister pack, while remembering her troubles, then scooping them all into her hand and swallowing. As the scene progresses, your character should develop a number of the symptoms typical of an antihistamine overdose, such as drowsiness, confusion, and hallucinations. You'll hook that reader, while avoiding getting a wrong drug-symptom combination.

Slang Terms

(Since terminology and slang terms change over time, further research is highly encouraged.)

Street names

DPH, drill, dryl, pink dreamz

Weaving the Plot

How is it used?

Antihistamine liquids and tablets are sold in packages labeled as allergy medicine, sleep aid, or cough syrup. The pills may come in safety blister packs or bulk bottles. The most distinctive of these are pink diphenhydramine pills. Other antihistamines are often white or yellow pills. Some antihistamines are available in combination cold tablets, but the multiple ingredients create a complex overdose picture and are best avoided for these scenes.

Don't have your character hallucinate after using an anti-itch cream.

Diphenhydramine is also available in creams used to stop itching. These don't absorb through the skin, however, so don't have your character hallucinate after rubbing some of the cream on an itchy rash. In medical facilities, diphenhydramine is also given as an injection, especially in urgent situations, such as during severe allergic reactions.

Now you try it

> **Writing Prompt #1** Write a scene as one of your own characters gets ready for work. Between a runny nose, constant sneezing, and itchy eyes, allergies are creating misery. With a big presentation to the company's boss due this morning, the character grabs a bottle of allergy pills and pours several pink pills out. Surely, a few extra pills will help hold off those pesky allergies through the presentation, right? (You'll continue this scene in Writing Prompt #2.)

How will my character act or feel?

At normal doses, your character will feel drowsy and have a slightly dry mouth. As the dose increases, more drowsiness can occur. With higher doses, severe sedation and confusion begin. Elderly characters or those drinking alcohol will have more pronounced antihistamine effects, even at normal doses, such as difficulty thinking and extreme drowsiness.

An overdose of diphenhydramine will cause many additional symptoms, including those described in the medical mnemonic. At first, your character will be drowsy, with some difficulty concentrating. She can be lucid enough to answer questions, but her words will become increasingly garbled from a mouth that's so dry it'll feel like it's stuffed with cotton balls. This can progress to include extreme sleepiness, blurry vision, confusion, irritability, and rambling thoughts. Her heart can be beating so fast that it feels as if it's shaking in place in her chest. She may vomit as her body tries to rid itself of the drug. If this happens, she could vomit enough to avoid serious symptoms. But if she's already become very drowsy or even unconscious, she risks choking on the vomit and either dying or suffering permanent disabilities from brain damage due to the lack of oxygen (see the appendix). If she doesn't pass out, her distress can get worse when the hallucinations begin. It's realistic for her to be agitated and physically combative, fighting anyone nearby as she desperately swipes at imaginary bugs crawling on her skin. Her skin should be flushed and hot from fever, but don't have her clothes damp from perspiring. High antihistamine doses block the body's ability to cool down through

Hallucinations of spiders crawling on the wall can realistically panic your character.

sweating. As her temperature soars, she can collapse from a seizure, her limbs jerking and foam dripping from her clenched mouth. The seizure can realistically stop, leaving her unconscious, or she could have a seizure that continues until medical help arrives. Without emergency medical care, your character can end up in a coma or she may die from a fatal, irregular heartbeat. And if she does survive, if her temperature isn't brought down rapidly enough, she can suffer brain damage.

Now you try it

> **Writing Prompt #2** Continue the scene from Writing Prompt #1. Your character has just started the presentation when symptoms from taking all those allergy pills begin. How does the presentation go?

How long will this drug affect my character?

Diphenhydramine takes about thirty minutes to begin causing sedation and dry mouth after it's swallowed. In higher doses, escalating symptoms will follow. Within two hours, your character should be struggling with serious symptoms that continue to worsen over yet another hour. If your character gets an injection of diphenhydramine, sedation can start within three to five minutes and, if it's a high dose, serious symptoms may appear as soon as fifteen to twenty minutes.

Effects from normally recommended doses last about three to four hours. With high (but not lethal) doses, a character's symptoms (like severe dry mouth, blurry vision, or grogginess) can slowly wear off, if she's lucky, over about four to six hours. She may even still be somewhat groggy the next day, however. But if you want her to have intense hallucinations or a temperature high enough to cause seizures, luck won't be on her side—if medical help doesn't arrive in time, she may realistically die.

Sample Scenario Kim finds her son passed out on the bathroom floor. She shakes him. "Frankie?" He moans. "Frankie, what happened?" He starts to answer, but drifts off, staring at the wall, his eyelids drooping. She places her hand on his forehead. *He's so hot! He must have a virus.* Frankie pushes her hand away, mumbling.

Now you try it

Writing Prompt #3 Finish the scene above, as Frankie begins to hallucinate from an overdose of antihistamines. What does he see? How does his mom react?

7

BATH SALTS

Brief History/Social Context

Looking for a drug to send a character into a crazed attack against terrifying hallucinations before landing in a psychiatric ward, restrained* to the bed? Bath salts are your answer. You may be wondering how the great smelling salts used for luxurious tub soaks can send your character into a psychotic frenzy. Well, they can't. These newer "bath salts" are actually a group of dangerous man-made chemicals called synthetic cathinones. Originally, they were designed to mimic the natural chemicals in the leaves of an African plant called khat (pronounced *cat*). For hundreds of years, khat leaves have been chewed in some cultures for increased alertness and energy. The *synthetic* chemicals, however, are much more powerful, with effects that are similar to combining an exaggerated high from cocaine stimulation with ecstasy-like hallucinations. Bath salts can also trigger uncontrollable rage, violence, horrifying hallucinations, self-harm, and psychotic breakdowns. And with the drug's pain-numbing effects and adrenaline bursts, your violent and hallucinating character can believably seem to have superhuman strength.

The main chemical in bath salts is known as MDPV (short for 3,4-methylenedioxypyrovalerone). But the content of bath salts isn't consistent, and they often contain a variety of chemical cousins to MDPV. In addition, batches have also been cut (diluted) with other drugs, including methamphetamine (meth), anesthetics, and Spice/K2 (see "Methamphetamine" in chapter 15 and "Spice/K2" in chapter 12). Because of this, symptoms from using bath salts are not consistent, making it hard for an

> **Bath salts can send your character into an uncontrollable rage with frightening hallucinations.**

emergency room physician to determine how to treat a patient, but fun for an author looking for some creative license.

The popularity of bath salts escalated in 2010 as a cheaper substitute for methamphetamine or cocaine and because of their hallucinogenic effects. At that time, raw ingredients from China began appearing in the US. By 2011, over twenty thousand emergency room visits listed bath salts as one of the causes for treatment. Because of growing use and the serious risks, legislation passed between 2011 and 2012 made synthetic cathinones illegal. Drug traffickers responded by changing their bath salt formulation to unregulated chemicals, making them technically still legal. Bath salts could then be promoted as a "legal high." Unfortunately, users mistakenly thought "legal" meant safe.

Does your story take place before 2011? It will be easy for your character to buy bath salts in drug paraphernalia stores, truck stops, and even convenience stores in small foil-wrapped packages with catchy names, like Cloud 9 or Vanilla Sky. For stories taking place after 2012, your character will buy his bath salts in packages labeled "not for human consumption" and advertised as jewelry cleaner, plant food, or phone screen cleaner, as the manufacturers found legal marketing loopholes.

As the chemicals used to make bath salts change, so do the unanticipated risks. For example, Flakka, a powerful designer bath salt, appeared in the US in 2015. It's been nicknamed the "Devil's Drug" or "Zombie Drug." Flakka causes frightening hallucinations, violent behavior, dangerous spikes in body temperature, and horrific self-harm (such as self-mutilation or jumping from a bridge). Flakka became so well-known that it was even included in the plot of the 2017 movie *Baywatch* as a new drug endangering the local community.

Devil's Drug causes frightening hallucinations and potential self-harm.

Bath salts have been used to cut (dilute) other street drugs, such as heroin. They have also been sold posing as other drugs, like ecstasy. So, your protagonist may unexpectedly become crazed and violent, not realizing his heroin was cut with bath salts. Bath salts have also been sold as a cheap substitute for popularly abused prescription stimulants, such as Ritalin or Adderall. This offers a potentially scary plot twist for a college student that's using stimulants to stay awake while studying for finals (see "Prescription Stimulants" in chapter 15). (*Restraint belts are very controversial and potentially dangerous with legal restrictions to their use. A medical professional critique partner is recommended to help guide the use of these in your scene.)*

Slang Terms

(Since terminology and slang terms change over time, further research is highly encouraged.)

Street names

arctic blast, aura, avalanche, bed dove, bliss, cloud 9, devil's drug, flakka, hurricane Charlie, lunar wave, MDPV, ocean snow, party powder, scarface, sextasy, vanilla sky, white dove, white lightening, white rush, white stallion, zombie drug (also refers to xylazine or tranq dope)

Weaving the Plot

How is it used?

The white to tan crystals or fine powder are usually snorted or sprinkled onto cigarettes (either marijuana or tobacco) to smoke. They can also be swallowed as capsules (eaten, popped), wrapped in a piece of paper to swallow (bombed), or injected (slammed). Sometimes, they're inserted vaginally or rectally.

Now you try it

> **Writing Prompt #1** Develop the backstory for one of your own characters that uses bath salts. What drove the decision to use them? How long ago did that occur? How has their use changed your character? (You will use this information in Writing Prompt #2.)

How will my character act or feel?

Keep in mind, that due to the wide variety of chemicals that could be in bath salts, it's hard to know what behaviors might occur. It's precisely the unknown possibility of extreme behavioral changes and the intensity of the symptoms that make bath salts tempting to use in a scene. The list of symptoms your character can suffer is almost nonending but can include crazed hallucinations, a painfully rapid heartbeat, seizures, and both dangerously high blood pressure and body temperature to name a few. For example, at first, your character can be enjoying the stimulant effects of his bath salts, becoming very chatty, sociable, and even happy, with a whole-body rush of energy. This can turn into agitation and his heart may race painfully in his chest. Want things to escalate? Consider adding disturbing symptoms, such as a panic attack or frightening hallucinations. He may see people whose faces melt and turn into terrifying creatures that are trying to attack him. Your character can become paranoid, believing someone wants to kidnap or harm him. Need seizures in your scene? They can be triggered in your character by his spike in body temperature. And dehydration will make that temperature soar even higher. Imagine your character wandering outside on an extremely hot day after snorting bath salts, then suddenly collapsing as his body convulses and foam drips from his mouth. Or maybe a character that's been partying all evening with bath salts forgot to drink fluids and falls to the floor seizing, his body burning up with fever. The fever can even be high enough to cause brain damage resulting in permanent disabilities (see the appendix). The high temperature combined with seizing can also lead to muscle breakdown that causes kidney failure and death. Use the search terms *hyperthermia* and *rhabdomyolysis* online for more information.

If extreme violence and psychotic behavior suit your plotting needs, bath salts can realistically send one of your characters into an uncontrollable rage, attacking anything and everyone nearby. He can become crazed, delusional, and dangerous. For example, his fever could make him believe his clothes are actually on fire. The flames that he sees will seem very real. This might cause him to rip off his clothes and violently attack others. He could also cause himself a life-threatening injury during this episode and not even realize it due to the pain-numbing effects of the drug.

Bath salts can send your character into a violent rage.

Looking for a great dramatic emergency room scene for that character high on bath salts? If he's crazed as he attempts to escape the horrifying hallucinations, he'll need to be sedated. But it won't be easy getting a shot into him as he violently thrashes about. He may even think the nurses and guards are really aliens trying to hurt him. It'll take several guards to hold him, while a nurse shoves the needle right through his pants into his butt (or thigh). But bath salts are so strong that a second dose will likely be needed. He'll continue his crazed struggle for several minutes longer—despite the common movie trope that drugs cause instant sedation—before his eyes finally droop then flutter closed, his arms flopping to his sides. The emergency team may put your character in restraints* (for his safety *and* theirs) until he's completely unconscious. Believably the sedatives won't work and stronger drugs might be needed to actually paralyze your character. If this is done, a breathing tube *must* be put into his throat or he'll die from the lack of oxygen. (Paralyzing drugs stop *all* muscles from working,

If your character is given a paralyzing drug he won't be able to breathe without the help of a ventilator.

including the breathing muscles.) Once unconscious, a transfer to the Intensive Care Unit (ICU) on a ventilator is realistic. Every twelve to twenty-four hours, the drugs will be stopped long enough to see if the aggression and hallucinations have stopped. If not, the drugs will be restarted, keeping the character unconscious. Even once the bath salts are finally out of his body, it could take over a week of heavy sedation before the psychotic effects wear off enough to allow him to be transferred to a psychiatric unit. This is a great opportunity for a well-crafted "all is lost" moment at the end of your second act. (*Restraint belts are very controversial and potentially dangerous with legal restrictions to their use. A medical professional critique partner is recommended to help guide the use of these in your scene.*)

Surprisingly, despite the horrible risks, the intense drug cravings caused by bath salts can lead to addiction. Then, if your character stops taking them he will suffer withdrawal, including body shakes (tremors), insomnia, paranoia, and depression along with the unbearable drug cravings.

With bath salts, your character may try to cut demons out of his body.

Death while high on bath salts can believably occur from a fatal stroke or heart attack during the adrenaline surges. In addition, life-threatening injury, such as running into traffic to escape hallucinations, can result in death.

As you can see, with bath salts, it's almost hard to make a scene that's too far-fetched. Real case reports include users physically attacking people, biting the paint off of vehicles, jumping from bridges, and self-inflicting life-threatening wounds (one person tried to cut demons out of his veins). Sadly, users have even begged police to kill them to end the terrifying experience.

Now you try it

> **Writing Prompt #2** Develop a scene from the point of view of your character from Writing Prompt #1 just as the high from the bath salts is wearing off. Where is the character? What happened during the high and how are those details revealed?

How long will this drug affect my character?

The rush from MDPV can start within five to ten minutes after snorting or about thirty minutes after swallowing the drug. Smoking or injecting bath salts brings rapid effects in just a minute or two. The energetic high and feeling of well-being can last three to four hours, but other side effects, such as agitation and a racing heart, can continue for eight hours or longer. Then, a hangover effect can last for another day or two. Intense hallucinations, aggression, violence, and psychotic behavior can occur at any time during the high and may last from several days to over a week.

PUTTING IT ALL TOGETHER

Sample Scenario #1 A disheveled man is yelling, beating his head against a cop car. Blood flows down his cheeks as a policeman grabs him. He slams his head into the officer, breaking away. The man yanks frantically at the car door as if trying to pull it off of the vehicle, then slams a fist through the window. Blood pours from his wounds as he continues pounding at the car until three officers tackle him to the ground. Thrashing on the pavement, he screams that demons are killing him.

Sample Scenario #2 Kai leans over, snorting a line on the tray. He smiles, letting the buzzy rush hit as he waits for the room to stop spinning. When it finally does, a jolt of energy pulses through him. Soon, he's talking loudly with his friends, his hands animated. He can't help himself—he keeps talking, pacing the floor, becoming more agitated. Then he notices his friends are staring at him strangely and whispering to each other.

Now you try it

Writing Prompt #3 Continue the scene with Kai (above) as his paranoia about his friends grows. Does he think they're plotting against him? Or do his friends morph into evil creatures that want to kill him? How does this scene end?

8

BODY PACKING

Just when you think you've seen everything, from snorting heroin to alcohol-soaked tampons, the world of body packing is a whole new kind of danger for your characters. In body packing, "mules" (smugglers) hide numerous small drug-filled packets in their body to avoid detection until reaching their destination. Popular drugs smuggled this way include cocaine, heroin, fentanyl, and methamphetamine just to name a few. Which drugs are smuggled varies based on many factors, including the geographic location, trends in use, and profitability. Powdered drugs have traditionally been smuggled, but liquid drugs are becoming more frequent since they're harder to detect with x-rays. Sometimes, drugs are smuggled as a paste. Newer drug packaging techniques and using specialized machines also make smuggling more difficult to detect.

With a variety of styles of body packing, you can decide just how your character tries to hide those drugs. "Packers" swallow the drug packets, whereas "shovers" hide them in body cavities. A "stuffer" is a smuggler who must suddenly swallow the packets or stuff them into a body cavity during urgent situations, such as imminent arrest. "Plugging" specifically refers to inserting the drug packets into the mule's rectum.

Who are these mules? They come from many walks of life—poor workers needing money, people in debt to a drug dealer, and even college students trying to make quick cash while returning from a vacation. Your character may be an adult, but teens and children are quite plausible as well. Some mules are paid to transport the drugs, but others are victims of human trafficking, forced to smuggle under the threat of physical harm or death.

So, just how many of these packets *will* you need to have your character hide? A lot more than you may think! There may be as many as one hundred packets, each containing several grams of drug, to tuck away. These packets, which are prone to breaking, were historically made by wrapping flimsy drug-filled condoms (sometimes multi-layered) with duct tape. Increasingly, packets are made using hollow pellets or sturdy, wax-coated plastics.

The many styles of body packing lend themselves to a wide variety of creative plots for writers.

How can you accurately depict swallowing so many packets? Your character can realistically be given an oily numbing liquid to coat his throat and ease the swallowing of all those packets. Then, to keep the packets from coming out with a bowel movement, he'll take an antidiarrhea drug (such as loperamide).

Wondering how he eventually *does* get all the packets out once reaching his destination? He'll need to take strong laxatives to force all the packets to come out. And, yes, he *will* have to make sure they *all* come out . . . so he's going to have to count them. Or the traffickers will have to count them. Either way, it doesn't paint a pretty picture.

As you can imagine, being a mule carries many risks. For stuffers, since their packets weren't originally designed to withstand swallowing or shoving, the drugs can leak out while inside the mule, releasing a deadly overdose. The packets can get lodged in a mule's throat or intestines (impaction). These stuck packets will then block anything else from getting through, such as food or water. The blocked intestines will make your character nauseous and his gut painfully swollen. He'll need emergency surgery to remove those stuck packets before they burst or his intestines tear and feces seep out, causing a life-threatening infection. Even if packets don't get stuck, mules always run the risk of the packets breaking at any time during smuggling or while those laxatives are forcing the gut to push them out—with a single packet containing enough drug to cause death.

Who will help your suffering character in these page-turning scenes? Maybe no one. Drug traffickers aren't too worried about getting medical help for mules who may be left to die. And the mule isn't likely to ask for help, fearing arrest for drug possession and smuggling. If your mule is being forced to smuggle, he may be unable to escape his trafficker's watch long enough to get help. Even if he manages to escape, death may occur before he can reach assistance. Some mules do ultimately arrive at an emergency room though, either on their own because of painful symptoms or brought by law enforcement.

Arrest is always a risk faced by these mules despite how hard they try to hide the drugs. For example, the packets can slip out of cavities accidentally, risking notice by the police. In this case, your mule would be prepared with backup supplies to rapidly repair and re-hide those packets. If your character is apprehended, an x-ray of his body will show his gut lined with numerous drug packets. Real-life examples of these images can be found using the keywords *body packing x-rays*. Researching these images online can help you understand why they're described using creative terms such as *tic-tac* sign or *double condom* sign. It's fascinating and frightening to see so many lethal packets inside a single human, knowing they could break at any moment.

> **Tension can be built using the many dangers body packers face, from arrest to lethal overdose.**

When writing a body packing scenario, the symptoms your character suffers from torn packets will vary greatly depending on the smuggled drug. A methamphetamine overdose will be very different from one from fentanyl (see "Methamphetamine" in chapter 15 and Fentanyl in chapter 13). Once any drug packets break, be prepared to kill off the character with severe and rapidly evolving symptoms. The character won't die instantly, but he isn't likely to make it to the next scene. If you do want your character to live, a plausible scenario is to have your desperate mule slip away from his captor just in time to get lifesaving help. Consider using this kind of scenario as a character's backstory—the driving force behind a desire to help others escape this dangerous lifestyle.

These scenarios will test your creativity, letting you combine the body packing information in this chapter with drug overdose symptoms found in the individual drug chapters.

PUTTING IT ALL TOGETHER

Sample Scenario I try not to look nervous. My stomach aches and I want to throw up. But Victor's sitting right next to me, making sure I don't screw up. He'll kill me if I don't get on that plane or if I tell *anyone* what he's making me do. The other girls look miserable too. I try to smile at Mya. She looks so scared. I see her eyes open wide, her hands suddenly gripping her belly. She leans over and pukes before falling to the floor. I try to get up, to go help, but Victor's hand firmly pushes me back into my chair. I watch, helplessly, as Mya's whole body starts shaking, foam dripping from her mouth.

Now you try it

Writing Prompt Write a scene using one of your own characters who's trying to get safely through airport security while body packing methamphetamine. How is the meth hidden? Decide if your character is arrested in security or makes it onto the flight only to have a few drug packets break after the plane takes off. Now what?

9

CLUB DRUGS

In the early 1900s, Mickey Finn, a Chicago bartender, was rumored to have drugged customers' drinks with a sedative, possibly chloral hydrate, to steal cash. This practice was eventually referred to as being "slipped a Mickey." The more modern term for this is referred to as "getting roofied," or having a drink "spiked." And, unfortunately, getting roofied remains fairly common, although today a drink may be spiked by anyone with a sinister motive in any setting, including bars, private parties, and dance clubs. In fact, the modern group of sedatives typically used to spike drinks have become known as "club drugs."

If you're developing a contemporary scene involving one of these drugs, you're not restricted to writing about robbery. On one end of the spectrum, your character may recreationally use a club drug to get high at a music festival or private party. On the other end, your story may be entering into the emotionally devastating world of date rape. Because of this latter use, these sedatives are also known as "date-rape drugs."

This chapter focuses on four popular club drugs: ecstasy, flunitrazepam (Rohypnol), ketamine, and GHB, although the list of drugs is immense and continues to expand.

Ecstasy/MDMA (Molly)

Brief History/Social Context

Ecstasy or MDMA (short for the chemical name 3,4-methylenedioxy-methamphentamine) was originally developed in the early 1900s by a German pharmaceutical company. Chemically, MDMA is a cousin to methamphetamine. In the 1970s, ecstasy was tested as a possible treatment for psychosis. By the early 1980s, abuse of ecstasy was already extremely popular, causing the Drug Enforcement Administration (DEA) to ban the drug. Ecstasy was again briefly studied in the 1990s to treat pain in terminally-ill patients and more recently as a potential treatment for Post-Traumatic Stress Disorder (PTSD). With its high potential for abuse and no currently accepted medical use, MDMA remains illegal in the US at this time.

Ecstasy is popular to abuse because it blends a light, happy mood with an amphetamine-like high (increased sociability, confidence, and energy) and the visual distortions of LSD (acid). But ecstasy has a dark side, including use as a date-rape drug, due to its ability to cause both sexual arousal and amnesia. Despite this, it remains a favorite party drug at clubs and raves (all night dance parties). It's also become increasingly accepted as a personal recreational drug and at private parties. For example, ecstasy has been hidden inside fancy appetizers at upscale cocktail parties to enhance socialization. Now *there's* a plot twist for you (see "Brieing" under "Other Terms" in this chapter).

> **Ecstasy gives your character LSD-like hallucinations with amphetamine-like energy.**

What kind of characters might use ecstasy? High schoolers, college students, young professionals, or high-society women are all good candidates.

Need a modern dangerous plot twist option? Although the nickname "Molly" originally referred to the pure synthetic molecule form of MDMA, ecstasy supplies are increasingly cut (diluted) with other drugs, such as cocaine, methamphetamine, or bath salts. Some drugs sold as ecstasy are actually bath salts or some other drug. In these cases, instead of the typical ecstasy high, your character may go down a darker, unexpected road. See those individual drug chapters for more specific details.

Slang Terms

(Since terminology and slang terms change over time, further research is highly encouraged.)

Street names

Adam, beans, biscuit, clarity, disco, E, E-bombs, Eve, go, hug drug, lover's speed, MD, MDMA, Molly, peace, rolls, Skittles, STP, X, XTC

Other terms

- Brieing: hiding ecstasy in pieces of soft cheese, such as brie, or small appetizers at social gatherings; the ecstasy helps decrease social inhibitions among party-goers.
- Booty bump: insertion of drugs into the rectum.

- Bumping: taking more than one pill at a time.
- Candy flipping: ecstasy and LSD taken together.
- Dipping (or dipsticking): sticking a finger into ecstasy powder, then licking it off the finger.
- Kitty flipping: ecstasy mixed with ketamine.
- Parachute: wrapping crushed ecstasy in tissue paper before swallowing in order to hide the bitter taste.
- Puddle (e-puddle): multiple ecstasy users together in a group, as in "They were in a puddle, rollin' hard."
- Rolling: when someone experiences ecstasy effects, as in "I was rollin' last night pretty good."
- Stacking: pressing two or three ecstasy tablets together to make a larger pill.
- Topping-up: taking more ecstasy before the effects of the first dose wears off to stay high longer.
- Trippin' balls: generically refers to being very high, as in "I took E last night and was trippin' balls, dude."

Weaving the Plot

How is it used?

Although ecstasy is available as capsules or a liquid, it's most well-known as brightly colored pills, often stamped with cartoon smiley faces or cartoon-like characters. Users may take one pill for the entire evening or a pill several times throughout the night. Seasoned users may choose to take several pills all at once. Some users binge on numerous pills in one night or throughout a weekend, while others just take ecstasy periodically, such as monthly. At some upscale parties, ecstasy pills have been hidden in appetizers, such as soft cheeses, to enhance the sociability of guests (see "Brieing" under "Other Terms" in this chapter).

Staying hydrated with electrolyte drinks instead of plain water can keep your character from having seizures.

Your character can snort crushed tablets as "bumps" from a table, the back of his hand, or from a holder, such as a pen cap. Despite the bitter taste, it's realistic for your character to lick ecstasy from his finger after dipping it into the powder. Since dehydration while on ecstasy is dangerous, he may ensure that he's drinking enough fluids by diluting the powder in bottled water ("Molly water"). To avoid the risk of seizures from drinking too much plain water, your character may mix the powder into an electrolyte drink, instead. However, mixing ecstasy into a strong flavored drink, like orange juice, will mask the bitter taste better. Another way to mask the bitter taste is by wrapping the ecstasy powder in a small bit of paper before swallowing ("parachuting"), but this delays the effects of ecstasy until the paper dissolves. Some users "cap" their own powder (fill capsules with ecstasy) to mask the bitterness.

Rarely, a crushed tablet might be smoked.

Now you try it

> **Writing Prompt #1** Develop the background for one of your own characters who uses ecstasy. Why would ecstasy be used? Is it used at parties or privately at home? How long has the character been doing this? (You'll use this background in Writing Prompt #2.)

How will my character act or feel?

Snorted ecstasy powder causes a burning sensation in the nose and bitter tasting nasal drips. But no matter how it's taken, your character will feel a euphoric high, pleasurable warmth, and an initial surge of energy, leaving him chatty. He'll be filled with happiness, peace, and a deep empathy for others. His experience will be very "chill" or mellow. Colors will seem more vibrant, color trails from lights will follow his gaze, and the world can appear "wavy." Because of an increased desire for touch, physical closeness, and hugging, he'll go to a social gathering to be around others while high. The intense sexual arousal from ecstasy can lead to a plot point all of its own. Hallucinations, which will be even more intense at higher doses, can leave your character interacting with imaginary people and fading in and out of reality.

The "come down" (when the high fades away), can leave a sad, empty, or depressed character missing the sheer joy and calm of the ecstasy high. On the other hand, an "afterglow," including a general sense of calm happiness, can last for days. Wanting to experience that high again eventually leads to chronic ecstasy use and the risk of withdrawal if he stops taking it. Withdrawal will leave your character depressed, irritable, and suffering insomnia, but it isn't usually lethal.

If your character *is* a regular ecstasy user, he'll know a few tricks to reduce side effects during a high, such as carrying a baby pacifier to avoid cracking teeth from the jaw clenching and teeth grinding caused by "rolling."

Ecstasy can fill
your character
with a deep sense
of empathy, love,
happiness, and
peace.

Ecstasy can also cause serious side effects. It stops the body from regulating temperature. Combining this effect with an active hot environment, such as on a packed dance floor, can lead to a dangerously high body temperature, seizures, and even heat stroke. These risks are reduced, if your character stays hydrated. But without enough hydration, the situation can become life-threatening. Emergency treatment will be needed to cool your feverish character's body down and avoid possible long-term brain damage (see the appendix) or death. On the other hand, drinking too many fluids, especially just water without electrolytes, will overdilute his blood, also causing seizures and possibly brain damage or death.

Is your character a long-time ecstasy abuser? The "magic" of the high may go away with repeated use, leaving him unable to get the satisfying high he craves. He can also suffer depression, insomnia, irritability, or memory loss.

Does your character take several doses in a short period of time? Rapid build-up of ecstasy in the body can become quickly toxic, causing seizures and possibly death.

Sadly, date-rape after being given MDMA is a real risk.

Now you try it

Writing Prompt #2 Write a scene using the background from Writing Prompt #1. Your character just swallowed some ecstasy pills. How will the character feel? Act? Interact with others?

How long will this drug affect my character?

The happy wave of peaceful euphoria starts in twenty to thirty minutes (slightly longer for parachuting) followed shortly by the sound and visual distortions and the intense sexual arousal. The experience can last about three to six hours. Even before the high starts, your character can lose the ability to mentally focus and may not understand conversations or events. Some effects will continue long after the high is gone. For example, since ecstasy changes the balance of brain chemicals, your character can suffer bouts of depression, insomnia, or anxiety attacks even weeks after the last dose.

Sample Scenario Parker meets his friends after work at a club. He's handed a bright tablet, swallows it, and heads to the packed dance floor. Soon, he's dancing to the most amazing music. When he moves his head, intensely colored streaks paint the air.

A friend hands him another pill and a baby pacifier. "Here, you're gonna need this."

Parker frowns. "Why?"

His friend smirks. "You'll see."

Parker swigs the pill down with a beer and keeps dancing. Soon, all around him, the lights and sounds are loudly buzzing. He pulls the girl he's dancing with closer, rubbing his hands over her arms— her skin is so amazing. She taps at his tightly clenched jaw, motioning to his pocket. Ah, so that's what the pacifier is for.

Now you try it

Writing Prompt #3 Continue the scene above. What happens if Parker forgets to stay hydrated and then walks a mile home on a hot summer evening while still rolling? Is anyone with him? How does this scene end?

FLUNITRAZEPAM (ROHYPNOL/ROOFIES)

Brief History/Social Context

If we're being honest, you're probably researching this drug to write a date-rape scene. Rohypnol (nicknamed "roofie") has become infamously known as a date-rape drug through movies and real life (see "A Note of Caution: Using Brand Names" in chapter 1). This is because the scariest effects of flunitrazepam include amnesia and decreased inhibitions, which leave a person vulnerable to sexual assault. Would you be surprised to know the chemical in Rohypnol, flunitrazepam, is legally sold in some countries to treat insomnia? In the US, however, flunitrazepam remains illegal due to its high rate of abuse driven by its ability to cause a rapid euphoria. It's also mixed with other drugs to enhance or balance their effects, such as boosting a heroin high or decreasing the agitation often caused by cocaine.

When your character's drink turns blue she should suspect roofies.

If you're developing a date-rape scenario, there's important history to note. For scenes set before 1997, the white, brand name tablets were tasteless, odorless, and colorless when dissolved in light-colored drinks. A victim would not know her drink was tainted. Because of safety concerns, the brand name manufacturer changed the formulation. Since 1997, the tablets have been oblong and green, with a blue-speckled dye core that turns light-colored drinks blue, alerting potential victims.

But there's a possible twist: *counterfeit* tablets don't contain the dye, nor do other drugs that are being sold a roofies, such as GHB and ecstasy. So, when your character at the bar comes back from the bathroom and feels comforted that her drink hasn't changed colors, she could be in more danger than she realizes.

Slang Terms

(Since terminology and slang terms change over time, further research is highly encouraged.)

Street names

circles, dos, floozies, forget pill, la rocha, lunch money drug, Mexican valium, pingus, R2, roach*, roach 2, roaches*, roachies, robutal, rochas dos, roofies, row-shay, wolfies (*also used to describe a leftover butt of a marijuana cigarette)

Other terms:

- Roofied: being unknowingly drugged by flunitrazepam or, increasingly, any club drug, as in "She was roofied."
- Spike: to mix drugs or alcohol into a drink, as in "He spiked her drink when she wasn't looking."

Weaving the Plot

How is it used?

Flunitrazepam tablets can be either swallowed or crushed and then snorted. They can be dissolved into the drink of an unsuspecting victim, an action referred to as "roofing" (by the perpetrator) or "getting roofied" (by the victim).

Now you try it

Writing Prompt #1 Write a scene from the point of view of a character planning to roofie a person at a bar. How does the character plan to do it? Is the motivation robbery? Sex? Kidnapping? (You'll continue this scene in Writing Prompt #2, with a surprise twist!)

How will my character act or feel?

Your character will feel a lightheaded euphoria with drowsiness and slowed responses, both mental and physical. Acting slightly drunk, confused, slurring her speech, or bumping into objects would be realistic. Her whole body may feel heavy. Hours can pass with her sitting in a blank stupor or she may pass out. The next day, the character may have a severe hangover, similar to drinking a lot of alcohol, with blocks of missing memory ("blackout").

Mixing roofies with alcohol can turn deadly. So, your antagonist could suddenly turn into a murderer if his victim already had several shots of vodka before he spiked her drink. *Now* what?

Your kidnapping scene can pivot to murder if roofies are combined with too much liquor.

Now you try it

Writing Prompt #2 Continue the scene from Writing Prompt #1, with the promised twist. Your character has just spiked his victim's drink. Create a disturbance at the bar, during which the drinks get switched, leaving your character sipping the wrong concoction. When is the mistake realized? How does this scene end?

How long will this drug affect my character?

The pills cause lightheadedness in about twenty minutes (slightly faster when mixed into a drink). Effects continue to get stronger, with dizzy, drunk-like feelings lasting up to eight hours, followed by a severe alcohol-like hangover for another twenty-four to forty-eight hours. Any missing memory usually doesn't return. If your character wants to prove she's been roofied, her urine needs to be tested within seventy-two hours of when she thinks she was drugged.

Sample Scenario Tate wakes up. His brain is foggy, his limbs heavy, his head pounding. He didn't drink *that* much, did he? He stumbles to the kitchen, managing to pour a cup of coffee, trying to recall last night. There was the beach party. Music. Frankie's lips turning blue from some pill—it looked ridiculous. The last thing Tate can remember is staring at one of those pills in his own palm.

*Due to their sensitive nature, example scenarios of date-rape will not be included here, but authors are welcome to develop their own scenes.

Now you try it

Writing Prompt #3 Continue the scenario above. Did Tate remember anything else he did at the party, such as taking the pill? What happens when he looks online and sees disturbing pictures from the party?

KETAMINE

Brief History/Social Context

Ketamine offers a wide variety of scenarios and backstories, from a character being treated for depression to one stuck in a nightmarish trip. Ketamine is a well-known drug of abuse, but you might be surprised to learn that it has been an extremely useful surgical anesthetic since its approval in 1970. In fact, it became instrumental in treating wounded soldiers on the Vietnam battlefields. After the war, it continued to be used as an anesthetic until it was temporarily replaced because of "emergence nightmares." This phenomenon caused patients that were waking from anesthesia to experience frightening hallucinations, sometimes lasting several hours and often requiring sedatives. Your character experiencing these nightmares as she wakes from surgery may try to crawl off the operating table, screaming, and lashing out in fear. Eventually, doctors learned how to control this phenomenon and ketamine anesthesia remains widely used today.

> Frightening nightmares can torment a character waking up from ketamine anesthesia.

Ketamine also has many other medical uses, including the treatment of severe pain in an emergency room and for uncontrollable seizures. More recently, ketamine has gained popularity for the treatment of depression and withdrawal. And emergency medical service (EMS) personnel use ketamine to help sedate combative, aggressive patients before transporting them to a hospital. However, the guidelines for ketamine use by EMS are being revised after a death in 2022. Before writing your scene, check for updated information online using the keywords *ketamine EMS guidelines*. In addition, each individual state department of health may publish their own EMS restrictions.

Ketamine is also highly abused. Some users seek the mellow, relaxed high and increased sociability offered by low ketamine doses. Others prefer the shorter hallucinogenic trips with ketamine compared to the longer trips associated with other psychedelics, like LSD (acid). Ketamine is also known as a dissociative hallucinogen, causing a complete disconnection from reality and an out-of-body experience that some users desire but others find frightening.

A delirious, combative character might be sedated with ketamine.

Ketamine can offer a number of ways to create trouble for your character. Abusing ketamine can cause him to suffer uncontrollable, frightening hallucinations. He can pass out and die during a hallucinogenic trip from choking on his own vomit. Or, if your character already has heart problems, ketamine could trigger a stroke or a heart attack. And if alcohol or heroin is being used with the ketamine, your character risks dying, as his breathing becomes dangerously slow or stops completely.

But don't try to save your character with an antidote. There isn't one for ketamine. Emergency medical personnel will only be able to treat his symptoms, such as his slowed breathing and seizures, until the drug wears off.

How will your character get ketamine? Because of abuse risks, this drug is very regulated. Generally, your character being treated for depression won't be able to get his doses from a local pharmacy. Instead, he'll receive them during supervised appointments in a ketamine clinic. However, there's a growing trend of at-home telemedicine treatment with real-time video-guided dose sessions. In these cases, the ketamine is shipped directly to the patient's home and each dose is taken during

Ketamine scenes can include a character experiencing a mellow relaxed high, an out-of-body experience, or LSD-like hallucinations.

a medically supervised video chat. Dispensing regulations may change, but currently a scene involving breaking into the corner drug store to steal ketamine is not realistic.

Despite tight distribution channels, diversion of prescription ketamine has increased. "Street" ketamine is also readily available and can be purchased at social events (like raves and dance clubs), through personal contacts, and even via social media apps. Homemade ketamine nasal sprays, from diverted or street supplies, are increasingly being used. These small bottles are ideal for your character to stash in his pocket and discreetly take bump-ups (small extra doses) throughout the night to maintain his sociable high. He could even bring a few extra bottles to sell.

Homemade ketamine nasal sprays will be easy for your character to get at a nightclub or rave.

Finally, like many drugs of abuse, illicit ketamine supplies have been increasingly tainted with other drugs, including cocaine, ecstasy, and even methamphetamine. In fact, with counterfeit drug supplies your character can't be sure that what he's using contains any ketamine at all, opening the door to a wide array of risks—and plot twists.

Slang Terms

(Since terminology and slang terms change over time, further research is highly encouraged.)

Street names

cat tranquilizer, cat valium, jet, jet K, ket, Kit Kat, k spray (nasal spray), liquid-E, regretamine, special K, super acid, super K, vitamin K

Other terms

- Bump: can refer to a dose or amount of ketamine, as in "I took a bump" or "I bought a bump."
- K-hole: the experience from a high dose of ketamine, including lack of awareness of surroundings, vivid hallucinations, and an out-of-body experience, as in "I dropped into the k-hole" or "I got lost in the k-hole."
- K-land: an experience from a lower dose of ketamine, with calm, mellow relaxation, increased sociability, and mild visual hallucinations.
- Trip sitter: someone who watches over a user during a trip to assure safety.

Weaving the Plot

How is it used?

Medically, ketamine is injected into either a vein (intravenous, IV) or a muscle (intramuscular, IM), or it may be given as a nasal spray.

Illicit ketamine may be a small, white to light brown granular powder (like salt), small white flakes, or a liquid. Increasingly, ketamine nasal spray is abused. Powdered ketamine is often packaged in small plastic baggies, capsules, or folded pieces of paper or aluminum. Your character can place the powder into lines (bumps) to snort or sprinkle it onto cigarettes (marijuana or tobacco) to smoke. The powder can also be diluted in warm water, then added to orange juice to mask the bitter taste. If the scene has your character injecting ketamine, consider having him stick the needle into his thigh instead of his vein (slamming). Slamming ketamine causes a fast, intense high and a disconcertingly rapid drop into the k-hole within seconds.

> **If your character slams ketamine, he may find himself dropping into the k-hole within seconds.**

Although ketamine is used by itself, it's not uncommon for it to be combined with alcohol, cocaine, or amphetamines. Users say ketamine can help revive a dying party.

Now you try it

> **Writing Prompt #1** Develop a scene using one of your own characters at a dance party. Someone offers ketamine and your character accepts. What drives your character to say yes? Has the character ever used ketamine before? Would this character choose to drink, snort, smoke, or inject it? (You'll continue this scene in Writing Prompt #2.)

How will my character act or feel?

Your character may take numerous small ketamine bumps throughout a social event using the nose spray or powder. He'll be able to remain conversational and maintain his relaxed sense of wellness, increased sociability, and happy dreamlike state. He might prefer using the nose spray since snorting the powder leaves a bitter aftertaste dripping down the throat. The spray bottles are also discreet.

As the ketamine buzzy high hits, even at moderately low doses, objects will seem to move slowly, dragging behind your character's vision as he turns his head and the world may have a wavy look to it. Taking another dose will magnify his high and cause mild body numbness, drowsiness, and slightly slurred speech. Now, when he turns his head, the dragging objects will have a distinct delay, leaving light trails as they move through the air. Midway through sentences, the character will lose his focus on the conversation and drift off. In addition, he might make dangerous decisions, not realizing his level of impairment.

Higher doses will drop your character "down the k-hole" into a world of distorted lights, sounds, and hallucinations. A loud static or ringing will fill his ears and physical numbness will leave him feeling disconnected from his body. During this time, shifts of space and time will seem real. For example, he may actually believe he's floating away from his body or riding on a roller coaster in space. His hallucinations, beautiful or frightening, will be vivid. He may even believe he has died.

In the k-hole, anything from drifting through space to horrifying hallucinations can occur.

During the character's trip, he might remain physically motionless, propped in a corner or staring at a wall. He may become frightened or agitated. He won't respond to questions or understand conversations, but may talk to people that don't exist. If his eyes are open, his friends will see his pupils darting back and forth.

Did the character drink ketamine? Add nausea and vomiting to his experience. Did he inject it into a vein? He'll drop into the k-hole within seconds. He might not even make it to his chair before falling to the floor, unconscious, the empty syringe lying next to him. Don't have him *instantly* drop to the ground, though. Give the reader a few sentences to stress as the character begins to realize how fast the k-hole is approaching before his world rapidly slips away. For example, the character's ears can suddenly fill with a loud buzzing and the room may look wavy. Then . . . boom! He's flying through space.

While high on ketamine, your character could become fatally injured.

With a k-hole trip, your character risks self-injury or death. Not only will he be unaware of his surroundings but his sense of pain will be dulled. Real cases have unfortunately involved users accidentally walking off of a roof or drowning in a bathtub while high.

The "come down" (loss of the high) with ketamine is a slow re-entrance into reality, leaving an afterglow, or sense of contentment, for several hours.

After the high, your character might recall having drifted away from his own body or having gained a deeper insight into life.

While k-land might be enjoyable at an energetic party, a quieter setting, such as a home or small, intimate party, is a better choice for a k-hole experience, since loud, stressful environments can trigger frightening hallucinations or bad trips. A designated trip sitter should monitor the experience to keep the character safe from dangers, such as behaving recklessly or choking on his own vomit.

A trip sitter is like a designated driver for ketamine users.

Is your character a chronic ketamine user? If he abruptly stops his ketamine habit, he'll become irritable, anxious, and not sleep well. The real world can begin to feel alien, leaving him depressed. But the ketamine world, which he finds more enjoyable, might tempt him back. He can develop memory problems or psychosis (incoherent speech, false beliefs, and delusions). A momentary vivid flashback to a previous trip can suddenly surprise him long after his last dose. And sharing needles with others injecting ketamine puts him at risk for diseases such as HIV (Human Immunodeficiency Virus) or hepatitis.

Now you try it

> **Writing Prompt #2** Continue the scene from Writing Prompt #1. Show the ketamine experience through the eyes and ears of your character. What's it like? How does the scene end?

How long will this drug affect my character?

Slowly injecting ketamine allows medical sedation without a high. But rapidly injecting ketamine (IV) or using the nasal spray causes a high within thirty seconds. When the powder is snorted or ketamine is injected into a muscle (IM), it can take a up to five minutes for the high to begin. The high from swallowing a dose takes even longer to start—up to twenty minutes. With small bumps, like in homemade nasal sprays, the come down from the high can occur within thirty minutes. After higher doses the hallucinations can continue for about an hour, but the other effects will last for several more hours (depending on the dose).

If the character experiences a flashback, it will last for only moments but will seem realistic.

Sample Scenario Casey wipes the powder from his nose and lets the calm wash over him. He tries to walk, stumbles, and sits back down laughing.

"Damn! I'm high as shit," he laughs and turns toward Amy, watching her stick a needle into her arm. Suddenly, a loud rush fills his ears and the room is gone. He's floating in darkness, drifting, feeling nothing. He seems to float forever. When his brain finally clears, he turns toward a noise. Amy's on the floor next to him, her lips blueish, vomit gurgling from her mouth.

Now you try it

Writing Prompt #3 Write a scene where a college student has a flashback of a frightening moment from a previous ketamine trip . . . in the middle of a class lecture. How do the other students or the professor react? What happens?

GHB (GAMMA HYDROXYBUTYRIC ACID)

Brief History/Social Context

Does your socially awkward character need a confidence booster at parties? Or are you crafting a more diabolical plot, leading to date rape or murder? Consider plotting with the drug GHB. Innocently enough, GHB (gamma hydroxybutyric acid) was originally sold as a dietary supplement in the US. It was believed to help with a wide variety of issues from insomnia to dementia. Weightlifters used it, claiming it offset the insomnia and restlessness caused by testosterone supplements, while bodybuilders believed it decreased body fat and increased muscle mass.

So how does this seemingly uninteresting dietary supplement give authors a page-turner? Well, GHB has long been a drug of abuse. The euphoria and decreased inhibitions it causes made it popular at raves as early as the 1990s. Over the last several years, GHB has spread to more mainstream use spurred by easy access and low cost. It's not uncommon to find it at music festivals, dance parties, and even private parties. Because GHB is odorless, colorless, and

A party scene can realistically include a dancefloor with teens high on GHB.

causes amnesia, it also has a history of use in date rape. In fact, sadly, GHB was used by a serial killer in the United Kingdom to rape and murder four young men.

GHB is difficult to safely dose—even small measuring errors can cause unexpectedly large (and potentially dangerous) changes in the effects. Because of the growing number of GHB-related overdoses, legislation was passed in 2000 making it a controlled substance. Undeterred, users turned to two unregulated GHB cousins with similar effects, GBL (gamma-butyrolactone) and BDO (1,4-butanediol). These chemicals were sold on the internet, labeled as "not for human consumption" and sold as cleaners (such as fish tank cleaner).

In 2006, legislation finally made internet sales of GHB and its chemical cousins illegal. But your character can *still* easily get GHB. It's made by clandestine labs and sold at bars, music festivals, raves, chemical sex parties (chemsex), and through social media platforms. GHB and its cousins can still be purchased online when sold as "cleaners." They're also falsely sold as ecstasy or roofies.

Medically, GHB is available as a prescription for very limited conditions, such as narcolepsy, but only through a strict oversight program and the doses can only be shipped by approved mail-order pharmacies. So, don't have your character plot a robbery at a local pharmacy to score some GHB.

Because these chemicals are made in clandestine labs, it's hard to ever know the purity or real content. Purity differences increase the risk of an overdose. So, when your character takes his usual GHB dose, he may get a lot more than he bargained for. This has led to an increase in homemade GHB, but the high sodium content in the recipe has led to nausea, vomiting, confusion, seizures, and even death.

> GHB will be easy for your character to buy through social media, at music festivals, or at parties.

Slang Terms

(Since terminology and slang terms change over time, further research is highly encouraged.)

Street names

easy lay, G, gamma-oh, geebs, George/Gina, Georgia home boy, grievous bodily harm, liquid E, liquid ecstasy, liquid X, the g's, and vitamin G

Other terms

- G-drops: drops of GHB.
- G-nap: falling asleep after taking GHB.
- G O'clock: time to take more GHB. Habitual users rely on an alarm clock to avoid the overdose risk associated with taking doses too frequently.
- Going under: overdosing, as in "She went under and didn't wake up."

Weaving the Plot

How is it used?

Liquid GHB is often carried in small medicine dropper bottles. Since the difference between a safe and dangerous dose is so small, the droppers are used for accurate measurement. Despite this concern, your character can plausibly buy GHB at a club or rave by the swig or capful. Some users will just swallow this concentrated GHB liquid, but because of the very salty, bitter, or soapy taste, many prefer to mix it into drinks to mask the flavor. This also helps avoid chemical irritation in the mouth. Sometimes GHB is sold in gelatin capsules, refillable dose bulbs, or pre-filled sealed straws to ensure an exact dose. Powdered GHB is rare, but can be snorted.

Does your character also use cocaine or Adderall? GHB can be used to soften the crash from these stimulants (see "Cocaine or Prescription Stimulants" in chapter 15).

Now you try it

> **Writing Prompt #1** Write a scene where a friend convinces your introverted, socially awkward character to take GHB before going to the school dance. (You'll continue writing this scene in Writing Prompt #2)

How will my character act or feel?

With GHB, as the dose increases so does the risk of more dangerous symptoms. At low "party doses," GHB will put your character into a really good mood, reduce his inhibitions, and leave him acting relaxed and socially confident. An introverted character will feel less socially isolated and be more talkative, giggly, and in control of life. Even at these low doses, it's credible for your character to experience euphoria and slight visual distortions or mild hallucinations. With higher doses GHB can cause drowsiness, staggering, clumsiness, nausea, and vomiting. The room may spin and the character can fade in and out of consciousness. GHB also causes sexual arousal, sometimes to the point of uncontrollable sexual desire. Together with a reduced ability to refuse sex and memory loss, rape is a real risk.

GHB can make your character become agitated and aggressive, starting fights for no reason. He can have a seizure, pass out from dangerously slow breathing, and possibly die. GHB can cause your character to fall into an abrupt coma only to wake on his own several hours later. It's very realistic to have him wake up in an emergency room after a short GHB coma and become combative with the medical staff who will need to sedate him for safety (his *and* theirs). Surprisingly, just a few hours later, he may be feeling good enough to be discharged from the hospital.

Your character can fall into an abrupt coma for several hours then suddenly awaken.

What about a character that's drinking plenty of vodka with his GHB? Liquor and GHB make a dangerous combination, causing GHB blood levels to rapidly build up. As the levels increase, your character's friends won't be able to wake him. He can believably collapse from a seizure and have foam dripping from his mouth. He may become comatose, completely stop breathing, and die.

New users are lured into continuing to take GHB because of the pleasurable experience and the lack of a hangover. Eventually, this leads to more frequent and higher doses, rapid addiction, and severe side effects.

Addiction can begin after just a few days of regular GHB. Starting just a few hours to a day after the character's last dose, he'll begin to suffer nausea, moodiness, jitteriness, palm sweating, confusion, yawning, and drowsiness— a warning that he's becoming addicted. If he walks away from GHB now, he'll suffer withdrawal symptoms for several days, but recover. But if the character continues taking GHB, he'll quickly notice that even as soon as two to three hours after a dose, he'll already be anxious, mentally foggy, and confused. Now, he'll be stuck in a cycle of dosing as often as every two hours to stave off withdrawal.

Need to make the character suffer more, as he slides toward rock bottom at the end of your second act? Once his addiction is very strong, let him run out of GHB and the money to get any more. For the next several days to two weeks, he can suffer tremors (like a shaking hand), nausea, vomiting, anxiety,

Even after just a few days of use, a character can suffer withdrawal symptoms from GHB.

insomnia, panic attacks, severe confusion, disorientation, and hallucinations. Without medical help during this stage of withdrawal, your character is in serious danger. Prolonged seizures can make it difficult for him to breathe, risking suffocation if he doesn't get help, such as with a ventilator, until the seizures stop. He can also suffer severe dehydration, dangerous muscle breakdown causing kidney damage, or psychotic episodes leading to self-injury or even death. High blood pressure surges can end in a stroke or heart attack. Fear of the misery of withdrawal will prompt your character to carry a bottle of GHB wherever he goes, if he can afford it. He'll also carry a timer for fear of overdosing from taking a dose too soon. When the alarm goes off, it's "G O'clock" and "safe" to take another dose.

What other realistic problems can your character have? Regular users mistakenly believe they're in control, unaware of their true level of impairment, and may make dangerous or bad choices. For example, your character may think it's safe to drive a car but end up in a serious crash.

Frequent doses cause GHB to build up in the body, increasing dangerous effects. Because of this, whether sitting on the beach or driving a car, the character can randomly pass out. When he awakens, he might find he has been robbed, sexually assaulted, or injured in a wreck.

> **Your character who suffered date rape needs to get to the ER within a few hours to be able to test for GHB.**

For date-rape scenarios, the victimized character must get to an emergency room within a few hours of the dose for GHB to show up on tests. (Don't write a scene using an at-home urine drug screen—they don't test for GHB.) Unfortunately, drug-induced amnesia will cause uncertainty about what actually happened, which may lead your character to delay getting medical help until it's too late for the urine test to work.

Over time, chronic abusers can develop *permanent* long-term effects, like limb-jerking, tremors, or severe insomnia.

Now you try it

> **Writing Prompt #2** Continue the scene from Writing Prompt #1. What happens at the dance? How does GHB make the character feel? Does the character take another dose to feel even better? What happens next?

How long will this drug affect my character?

The high starts within twenty to thirty minutes with the effects lasting three to five hours. Even in high doses, the effects may disappear within six hours (if no alcohol was consumed and no dangerous symptoms have started). In chronic abusers, GHB will only last two to three hours.

PUTTING IT ALL TOGETHER

Sample Scenario Elena laughs into her phone, then pauses, smiling at her mom in the kitchen. She turns back to her call. "Uhhh . . ." she hesitates, "so . . . is Gina gonna be there?" When Elena finally hangs up, her mom turns to her, an eyebrow cocked, her arms folded across her chest.
"I've never heard you mention Gina."

Now you try it

Writing Prompt #3 Write a scene for a character who decides to not bother measuring GHB anymore. At a party, the character free-pours GHB into several drinks throughout the evening. Decide how this scene will progress. What happens to the character?

Writing Prompt #4 For several days, your character has been partying with friends, taking GHB every few hours to stay high. Write a scene where the character has run out of money and no one is willing to share their GHB for free. Does withdrawal begin? What happens next?

10

HALLUCINOGENS

All hallucinogens, from natural plant extracts to synthetic chemicals, have one thing in common: they can create an escape from reality by distorting the senses. Your character can hear colors, see visual distortions of objects or people, lose the sense of time, and lack an awareness of pain. In addition, some hallucinogens can cause out-of-body experiences or even addiction.

Story possibilities go far beyond the trope of hippies high on LSD (acid). Your stressed high-level executive protagonist may use LSD to escape the realities of life for a while. Maybe a character's hallucinating from his cough syrup abuse. Or you can craft a more sinister plot, where your character believes she's losing her mind, not realizing her favorite sister is secretly slipping hallucinogenic mushrooms into her food in a diabolical plan to take over the family fortune.

There are so many plot options to consider!

With countless hallucinogens and a growing number becoming increasingly popular, this chapter focuses on a few of the more well-known drugs, including LSD, magic mushrooms, peyote (mescaline), and dextromethorphan (DXM). Two others, ecstasy and ketamine, are discussed in chapter 9.

LSD (D-Lysergic Acid Diethylamide, "Acid")

Brief History/Social Context

The effects of LSD were accidentally discovered by Dr. Albert Hofmann while hallucinating on a bike ride after being exposed to the drug in his lab. He originally developed LSD for potential medical use in the 1930s. A few years later, he experienced mild psychedelic effects after getting a small amount of LSD on his finger. And this is where his story becomes famous: a few days later, he *intentionally* took LSD, then, on his bike ride home, the hallucinations started. Imagine *that* bike ride! His experience became so famous that "Bicycle Day" is still celebrated every April 19 to commemorate his discovery. Proponents of LSD are quick to note that Hofmann electively took small doses of LSD regularly for the rest of his life.

Albert Hofmann unexpectedly discovered LSD hallucinations while riding his bike.

Hofmann extracted this odorless, colorless, bitter drug from a fungus. *LSD* stands for the full chemical name: D-lysergic acid diethylamide, but it's more famously known as "acid." During the 1950s and 1960s, Delysid (LSD-25) was used in psychotherapy research for the treatment of addiction and some mood disorders. But what started out as an intriguing, "trippy" medical treatment unfortunately became a major drug of abuse by the 1960s, due to its ability to cause hallucinations and what users called "an awakening of the mind." Subsequently, in the mid-1960s, the Food and Drug Administration (FDA) made LSD illegal in the US, bringing research to a halt and reducing access to recreational use. Recently, both recreational use and research into medical treatments with LSD are on the rise again in what is being called a "psychedelic renaissance."

While LSD remains popular for experiencing hallucinogenic "trips," it's also gained broader use in much smaller doses as consumers sought alternate interventions for depression and addiction. These "microdoses," when used correctly, are too small to cause hallucinations and are actively being studied for possible medical use. Among college students and young business workers, the use of microdoses of LSD (and other hallucinogens) has become popular with the belief that they increase energy and creativity, thereby enhancing the ability to remain competitive. Another growing trend called "psychedelic parenting" involves the use of these microdoses to reduce the stress of parenting.

Psychedelic parenting offers an interesting habit for a character.

Despite the potential medical benefits of LSD, there are also real dangers, including frightening hallucinations, impaired judgment leading to deadly injury, and psychosis. Emergency medical calls related to LSD experiences often involve people that are suffering severe anxiety, panic attacks, or confusion related to not having the proper "set and setting" before taking the dose. Set and setting refer to preparing a proper mental state and choosing an appropriate location for a calm and thoughtful experience. Poor set and setting preparation is also associated with frightening hallucinations and bad trips. Flashbacks (suddenly reliving a previous trip) can happen long after the last dose of LSD. In fact, in Denmark, patients treated with LSD were legally compensated after suffering long-term harm, including debilitating flashbacks. In addition, several suicides, suicide attempts, and one homicide occurred in the LSD treated patients, although the relationship to the treatment has been debated.

While death from actions during an LSD trip can occur, it's not realistic to have your character die simply from taking an overdose of this hallucinogen. Yes, a very high dose can cause an emotionally traumatic, extremely prolonged trip. But physical death from large doses has rarely been reported. However, LSD supplies have increasingly been tainted with other dangerous drugs. Your character could accidentally get acid tainted with NBOMe, a potent designer drug. Even very small doses of NBOMe can cause agitation, severe anxiety, hallucinations, panic, fast heart rates, high blood pressure, organ failure, and death.

Slang Terms

(Since terminology and slang terms change over time, further research is highly encouraged.)

Street names

acid, battery acid, blotter acid, dots or microdots (the tablets), loony toons, Lucy, mellow yellow, window pane (especially when in gelatin), zen

Other terms

- Blotter: a sheet of blotter paper dipped into LSD and perforated into multiple doses (tabs or hits), each with a colorful picture, similar to a sheet of stamps. Also called a sheet.
- Candy flipping: taking LSD with ecstasy (MDMA, "X"); LSD is often taken first, followed by MDMA within a few hours, as in "She brought some X and we went candy flippin' last night."
- Dropping acid: taking LSD, as in "I dropped a hit of acid."
- Hit(s): dose(s), as in "I did ten hits."
- Journey: refers to the LSD experience. Also see trip.
- Microdosing: using doses of psychedelics, such as LSD, that are too small to cause hallucinations but are believed to improve thought, creativity, depression, and even the mental fogginess from traumatic brain injury.
- Microdots: small pills containing LSD. Sometimes just "dots."
- Sheet: a sheet of blotter paper dipped into LSD and perforated into multiple doses (tabs or hits), each with a colorful picture, similar to a sheet of stamps. Also called a blotter.

- Stamp: an individual square from a dosing blotter, as in "I ate two stamps."
- Ten-strip: a strip of blotter paper containing ten hits of acid, as in "I did a 10-strip last week and was trippin' balls for 16 hours."
- Trip, tripping: the visual and auditory experience from LSD. Also called a journey.
- Window pane: colored gelatin sheet containing LSD typically divided into individual dosing squares called tabs or hits.

Weaving the Plot

How is it used?

Liquid LSD is often dropped onto a carrier, such as a sugar cube or gummy candy, to suck or swallow. Perforated colored blotter paper may be dipped into LSD liquid, dried, and then ripped into individual dosing squares. Gelatin sheets made with LSD are also cut into individual doses. The doses are held in the mouth or under the tongue to suck on before swallowing, causing a faster and more intense high than if just swallowed. When sold in a dropper bottle ("breath drops"), LSD is dropped directly onto or under the tongue. The LSD itself is tasteless with any flavor coming from the paper, candy, or gelatin carrying the drug.

Microdosing must be individualized, since the amount of LSD that causes hallucinations is different for each person. To decide the right dose, generally, a very low dose is initially taken and slowly increased until the first visual or sound alterations are noticed. The right dose, then, is just below that amount. Finding that right dose takes trial and error, lending itself to an interesting plot twist! But don't have your character taking these mini-LSD doses every day, since that can cause a condition called tolerance, where higher doses are needed to get the desired effect. Many dosing schedules are used, but they often include taking a dose daily for anywhere from one to several days, followed by some type of a "drug holiday." This drug-free period is said to take advantage of ongoing drug effects (the "afterglow") without developing tolerance. So your character might even just take microdoses of LSD only on the weekend and still feel emotionally uplifted throughout the week.

Your character might have to experiment to get the right microdose, creating an interesting plot twist.

LSD may also be "stacked" with other hallucinogens (and some vitamins) to get a combination of effects from various drugs.

Now you try it

Writing Prompt #1 Develop a scene with one of your characters at a party where LSD is being shared. What's the motivation to take it? A sense of adventure? Or has your character used it before? (You'll continue this scene in Writing Prompt #2.)

How will my character act or feel?

LSD trips are said to be a more intellectually enlightening than the more emotional experiences of hallucinogenic mushrooms. However, the effects of LSD on each person are unpredictable and can be impacted by a person's emotional state, recent life events, and the location where the hit (dose) is taken.

For traditional hallucinogenic doses of LSD, your character will have no control over the hallucinations (trip). The "come up" of the high, with visual and mood changes, will begin shortly after taking LSD and continue to increase. Colors and lights will become brighter and more vibrant to her. The room may seem to undulate or vibrate with colors changing and pulsing like a kaleidoscope. Her senses can get mixed, such as "hearing colors" or "seeing sounds." People and objects become warped and distorted, morphing from one look to another in hard-to-describe ways. To your character, people may look like glowing angels or beings from another world. Emotionally, she may have developed an indescribably pure love for others and believe she's gained intense insight into herself.

Seeing sounds and hearing colors can intensify your character's LSD trip.

Repressed memories, life stresses, or depression can turn your character's pleasant LSD experience into a "bad trip." This can also occur if she panics or becomes anxious during the experience, especially if there isn't a trip sitter to guide her back to a calm state. In a bad trip, your character might believe she's truly losing her mind or she may have frightening hallucinations, such as being chased by monsters. She might see shadows of evil people lurking in corners. Or she can wake up to find herself handcuffed to a gurney in an emergency room after having tried to attack those monsters, who turned out to actually be police officers.

Other dangers with tripping on LSD can include the risk of personal harm, such as walking out into traffic or being unaware of a severe injury due to the pain-blunting effects of the drug. High doses can also cause an extremely prolonged trip or lead to a psychotic breakdown.

Microdoses of LSD will need to be portrayed differently in your scenarios. Unless your character takes the wrong dose, it would not be realistic for her to experience halluci-

Depression or anxiety can set your character up for a bad trip.

nations. The world may seem to shimmer, but don't have her tripping. Your character may believe she's happier, more energetic, and more sociable. Is your character into psychedelic parenting? She can be portrayed as believing the drug has made it easier to cope with the daily pressures of parenthood.

Don't plan to develop a character that's addicted to LSD, however. A typical physical addiction to this drug is rare. A *psychological* addiction to the hallucinations or the mind-altering effects can be a realistic character flaw, however, especially if she begins to prefer the psychedelic world over her own.

Now you try it

> **Writing Prompt #2** Continue the scene from Writing Prompt #1. How intense of an experience do you want your character to have? Will it be a mild, happy experience? Will the character have beautiful hallucinations? Or a frightening trip?

How long will this drug affect my character?

The first signs that an LSD trip is starting may simply be subtle changes to the hues of colors or slightly shimmering objects. This can start within fifteen to sixty minutes and accelerate from there. Your character won't be able to control the length of a trip, though, which can last from six to as long as twelve hours, depending on the dose. Once the hallucinations begin to subside, she still won't feel quite normal for several more hours. She'll be tired and dehydrated from not drinking fluids during the lengthy trip. After the high completely wears off, she can suffer mild depression for a day or two, followed by several days or weeks of a lighter, happier mood with a better outlook on life (although not everyone experiences this).

Microdosing LSD creates an afterglow effect that lasts for several days after a dose, during which mood and energy reportedly continue to improve.

Prefer a scarier after-trip effect? A momentary flashback can happen days or months after the last dose, leaving your character frightened and feeling out of control—and can make a fun scene to explore. Flashbacks can be triggered by severe life stresses or fatigue among many other things.

Sample Scenario #1 She wiped the tears off her cheeks, but winced as she brushed across her tender jaw where his fist had landed. As she meandered through the park, her fingers reached into her pocket pulling out another bright yellow square. She popped it under her tongue. By the time she reached the pier, the water rippled with pulses of the most beautiful bright blue she'd ever seen. She dipped her toes into the lake, making more pulsing swirls. Above her, blinding white clouds swirled against the sky. Birds flew by, leaving light trails behind them. Then one of the birds turned its head toward her and smiled. Her heart began racing as she was filled with dread. When she looked down at her foot in the lake, the watery swirls around her toes had turned to blood and the whole lake was dark red. As she got up to run away, she heard laughing and looked up to see the birds perched on a tree, staring at her, taunting her. She scrambled to get away just as the birds began to chase her.

Sample Scenario #2 Ken smiles, staring at the vibrant hues of orange and red pulsing from the poster on his wall. Justice sits next to him, glowing like an angel. He touches her arm and feels the pulses of energy move from her through him. He knows now. He understands. She is pure, she is absolute, she *is* love.

Now you try it

Writing Prompt #3 Write a scene for a parent that took a micro dose of LSD before taking the kids to the grocery store. The twist? Your character made a mistake and took a bit too much. How will that trip to the store go? What will the kids (or the other shoppers) think? Have some fun with this one!

MAGIC MUSHROOMS

Brief History/Social Context

If you're looking for a psychedelic drug but LSD doesn't quite fit your character, then "magic mushrooms" may be an option. Hundreds of mushroom plants contain psilocybin, one of the main drugs considered responsible for the mind-altering effects from magic mushrooms. These plants are found across parts of Mexico, South America, and the United States. The chemical psilocybin remains illegal in the US, although a growing number of cities have decriminalized possession of the actual mushrooms. Two states recently legalized psilocybin mushrooms and details about the restrictions for medical or personal use are still evolving. In the meantime, the Food and Drug Administration (FDA) is considering approval of psilocybin for certain uses, such as depression, withdrawal, and posttraumatic stress disorder, pending additional medical studies. However, this will most likely include some form of medically supervised treatment in a clinical setting using a licensed facilitator to guide the experience. It's not likely that one of your characters will be able to get psilocybin mushrooms from a local pharmacy any time soon. As quickly as the laws are changing, for any contemporary manuscript, it's recommended to verify the legal status of hallucinogenic mushrooms in your story setting. For the most up-to-date status, good sources include the Department of Health websites for various states.

The rapidly changing legal status of magic mushrooms may impact how you approach your plot.

Hallucinogenic mushrooms have been used for thousands of years by spiritual healers and in religious ceremonies, especially within indigenous cultures. However, like LSD, magic mushrooms became famous in the US during the psychedelic revolution of the 1960s for their ability to cause hallucinogenic trips, a perceived awakening of the mind, and a deeper understanding of life. These mushrooms are still used today and are becoming more widely accepted.

Authors of contemporary fiction can believably include mind-altering magic mushroom experiences in a wide variety of settings, from a college dorm to dance clubs to the character's home. Some users take the mushrooms for an enlightening hallucinogenic journey, while others use "heroic doses" (very high doses) that are said to create indescribably profound trips. But your modern-day character may not even want to experience hallucinations. Instead, she may take part in the newest trend that involves taking doses that are too small to cause sensory distortions. These "microdoses" are said to decrease anxiety, tobacco addiction, alcohol addiction, and depression. Mushrooms are even advocated by some users as inexpensive alternatives to

A character can plausibly take magic mushrooms without having hallucinations.

formal depression treatment programs since they cost only a few dollars compared to the hundreds or thousands of dollars for the programs and their related prescription drugs, such as ketamine.

The microdosing trend has also been adopted by some young professionals and students who believe it increases creativity, energy, mental sharpness, and their ability to remain competitive in their field. Another new microdosing trend, called "psychedelic parenting," involves parents taking tiny magic mushroom doses believing they reduce stress and improve coping mechanisms, allowing them to be better parents.

Your character may be into psychedelic parenting.

The medical use of magic mushrooms is still very controversial. Medical studies are ongoing for the treatment of mood and addiction disorders with some early positive results, but bigger studies examining the potential uses and risks with psychedelic mushrooms are still pending. How does that impact you as an author? While you can realistically portray your character privately using magic mushrooms for depression or to reduce parenting stress, it would not be realistic to have a doctor prescribe them. At least not yet. As new information comes out, that may change. But for now, the doses are very experimental.

While magic mushrooms sound pretty uplifting, your character's enlightening journey can turn into an unpleasant, frightening trip. This can occur at higher doses or if she's in a loud or stressful environment. Users recommend taking mushrooms with an unstressed, focused mindset and in a calm, decluttered place to reduce the risk of a bad experience. A trip sitter would also be important to help guide your character through any unpleasant feelings and avoid the experience turning into a bad trip, which can include deep grief, anxiety, frightening hallucinations, fear of insanity, paranoia, panic attacks, and even psychotic behavior. If your character's trip *does* turn bad, she can realistically find herself running from a fire-breathing dragon or see monsters coming out of the floor. Without a trip sitter, impaired judgement, such as believing the mushroom effects have ended when they haven't, can lead your character to make dangerous choices, such as driving a car, leading to injury or death.

A flashback can occur at the most inopportune time in your character's life.

Months after your character's trip, she can find herself in the middle of a flashback, momentarily reliving a previous trip, good or bad. Now *that* sounds like a fun scene to explore.

How will your character get the magic mushrooms? That can be a challenge. Your microdosing mom isn't going to find them in the local grocery store—at least not yet. But a surprising number of illicit drugs are readily purchased on certain social media apps, sometimes complete with delivery. It's more likely, though, that a parent would be exposed to the concept of magic mushrooms by another parent who already microdoses and shares their own supply. Others find sources from acquaintances or at music festivals. In some states, retailers are exploring the legal loophole of selling "psilocybin-like" mushrooms, which contain hallucinogenic chemicals that are not yet illegal. In states that are moving to legalize magic mushrooms, they may soon be available in dispensaries, similar to medical marijuana.

Knowing a safe source would be crucial since there are risks when buying magic mushrooms. There can be little certainty of the actual strength or content when buying from unknown sources. For example, some "magic mushrooms" are actually just grocery store mushrooms that have been laced with LSD (acid) or other drugs. And unless your character *really* knows his plants, picking wild-growing mushrooms can end badly as there are many look alike plants, including poisonous varieties. Pick the wrong mushroom and your character could die.

Picking the wrong wild mushroom can be deadly for your character.

With the difficulty of having reliable sources, some users grow their own magic mushrooms. The spores are legal to purchase since they don't contain psilocybin, which is created as the plant matures. Kits are readily available online, complete with instructions for growing those little spores into a psychedelic mushroom supply. With evolving laws, legally growing psilocybin mushrooms at home may even become trendy. Imagine your quirky, famous murder investigator that solves crimes by day and tends to his magic mushroom garden at night.

Slang Terms

(Since terminology and slang terms change over time, further research is highly encouraged.)

Street names

boomers, buttons, gold's flesh, magic mushrooms, musk, pizza toppings, sacred shrooms, shrooms, silly putty, simple Simon

Other terms

- Come-up: the start of the trip or experience.
- Flush: a harvested crop of mushrooms.
- Hero dose: a large dose of magic mushrooms taken by some experienced users looking for a deep introspective experience.
- Hippie flip: taking MDMA with hallucinogenic mushrooms.
- Journey: refers to the experience while on the magic mushrooms. Also called a trip.
- Microdoses: very small doses of hallucinogens believed to clarify thought, improve creativity, and reduce depression without hallucinogenic effects.
- Psychedelic parenting: the trend of taking a microdose of magic mushrooms with the belief that it will reduce parenting stress or relieve post-partum depression.
- Stacking: the practice of taking other hallucinogens and supplements together with psilocybin mushrooms. The blend is believed to create complimentary effects.

Weaving the Plot

How is it used?

Psilocybin mushrooms are taken in such a wide variety of ways that it can be difficult to list them all. A few of the more popular methods are described here. Because of their extremely bitter, earthy taste, the mushrooms are often coated in small amounts of peanut butter or chocolate, or mixed into other foods. So that scene where a character is handed a spinach smoothie or a peanut butter sandwich "with an extra kick" can pivot the story in a whole new direction. Some users bite into the whole mushroom, despite the bitterness, but this can easily lead to a dose error. Capsules or teas from ground dried mushrooms are popular. A more creative drink known as lemon tek uses concentrated lemon juice thought to speed the chemical conversion of ground mushrooms into their active form. Because of this, lemon tek is said to create a faster, more intense high. Even chewable gummies are made from magic mushrooms. Imagine one of your character's kids accidentally eating those!

How much magic mushroom should you have your character take? It really depends on where your scene is headed. In general, if your character is only taking a little bit, he can stay mentally sharp and socially engaged with only small visual distortions. This character may swallow a couple of capsules or chew a mushroom gummy before going to work. Moderate to high doses will cause progressively more intense psychedelic hallucinations and emotional effects.

There's no specific microdose because the dose that causes hallucinations is different for each person and can vary with batch potency. So, the right amount to take must be individualized by starting with a small dose and slowly increasing it until visual or auditory disturbances begin. The right dose, then, is just below that. Obviously, this process takes trial and error lending itself to an interesting scenario! But don't have your character taking these mini-mushroom doses daily, since this can cause tolerance, where higher and higher doses are needed to get the desired effect. Doses are usually taken daily for one to several days in a row, followed by a "drug holiday," to avoid tolerance. This also takes advantage of the afterglow, during which subtle effects, such as elevated mood, continue.

> **Finding the right microdose will be a bit of an experiment—that could go wrong—for your character.**

Psilocybin mushrooms may also be "stacked" with other hallucinogens (and some vitamins) to get a blend of effects.

Now you try it

> **Writing Prompt #1** Develop the background for one of your own characters who's planning to take magic mushrooms. What's the character's motivation to do this? Has the character done this before? (You'll use this background in Writing Prompt #2.)

How will my character will act or feel?

There are some consistent and some very individualized experiences reported with hallucinogenic mushrooms. Many users describe deeply emotional journeys, seeing unexpected beauty in one's surroundings, and a deep awakening of the mind. But the experience can be impacted by the dose, the mindset of the user, and the atmosphere of the setting where the trip takes place. A serene setting may create an enjoyable, relaxing, introspective trip. A loud, stressful setting or an anxious mind can lead to an unexpectedly frightening experience.

In general, nausea and vomiting can plague your character during the first hour after taking hallucinogenic mushrooms, especially if food was recently eaten. An empty stomach will cause less stomach upset. So, some users prepare for a trip by fasting for a period beforehand. After about thirty minutes to an hour, your character will notice sensory changes with the "come up." Sounds may take on a new quality. Colors may become more vivid. The visual hallucinations are usually distortions of reality, such as shifting geometric patterns on a quilt, as opposed to seeing things that don't exist.

With microdoses your character can be depicted as having an uplifted mood, increased energy, and a clear mind. She may describe the world as a little sparkly or glowing. But don't plan on her having hallucinations, unless, of course, you intend for her to get the wrong dose.

At low doses, the character can have fairly normal social interactions with minor changes to sights and sounds. So, in class, at work, or in the nightclub, she may see soft color-trails streaking behind lights or hear unusual depth to sounds in her slightly dreamy world. She might find herself laughing or giggling a lot. Objects or people may look deeply, indescribably beautiful.

Psilocybin experiences vary widely, depending on the dose, person, state of mind, and surroundings.

As the dose increases, more intense distortions of color and sound will occur. Objects may seem to vibrate or move. Depth perception and spatial understanding will be confused—something that looks small because it's actually far away may be perceived as a nearby miniature. Strong emotions can overtake the character, from laughing to crying, triggered by sights, sounds, or memories.

Your character can realistically experience a true psychedelic trip at high doses, including the blending of colors, sights, and sounds as if she's looking through an audible kaleidoscope. The world can look beautifully mystical and surreal and she won't be able to tell reality from fantasy. She might also feel weak, drowsy, and clumsy. After the journey, your character can believe that she's gained a deeper understanding of life and the world around her. She may have an afterglow, with a happier, lighter mood for several days to weeks.

Planning a bad trip for the character? There are several believable ways to turn a calm journey into a frightening experience. Becoming stressed or worried about the trip can cause her to suffer a panic attack with a racing heart and profuse sweating. Disturbing hallucinations can be triggered by recent sad experiences, such as a death in the family or repressed bad memories. She can develop extreme paranoia, believing others are conspiring against her or that they're evil demons. She may also believe she's losing her mind. Later, your character can have trouble forgetting those disturbing

Bad trips can be triggered by stressful life events or repressed memories.

visions and may even have a psychotic breakdown. Finally, magic mushrooms carry the risk of uncovering or worsening certain mental illnesses, such as schizophrenia.

If you need an even darker twist, bad choices, such driving a car or walking into traffic while under the influence of hallucinogenic mushrooms can lead to deadly consequences. This is especially true if the character doesn't have a trip sitter to guide her away from dangers.

Your character should not get physically addicted to magic mushrooms.

If you want your character to become addicted to mushrooms, make it a *psychological* addiction, not physical. Don't have your character develop physical withdrawal symptoms, like cravings or seizures. These are not realistic with psilocybin mushrooms. But she *can* get to the point where she thinks she can't emotionally handle life's stresses and emotions without the mushrooms.

Now you try it

> **Writing Prompt #2** Using the background from Writing Prompt #1, write a scene as your character takes the mushrooms. Show the experience through your character's eyes.

How long will this drug affect my character?

Effects start in about thirty minutes to an hour and increase over the next one to two hours. A low to moderate dose can cause a trip that lasts four to six hours, while a heroic dose can cause effects for six to eight hours. The afterglow of lighter mood and happier outlook can last several days longer. Microdosing effects can last for one to several days after the last dose.

PUTTING IT ALL TOGETHER

> **Sample Scenario #1** Avery sips the bitter tea at the campfire, watching quietly as the flames turn purple and green, then lick up at the clouds in the darkening sky. When he closes his eyes, a colorful kaleidoscope swirls before him. When he opens them again, tears well up in his eyes as the bright stars pulse against a pitch-black sky. He's never seen anything so utterly beautiful.

Now you try it

> **Writing Prompt #3** Continue the scene with Elena, above. What happened at the audition when the magic mushroom-filled kale milkshake started taking effect?
>
> **Writing Prompt #4** Write a scene for a character who's at the circus with her three kids. The twist? She accidentally took a few too many of her magic mushroom gummies before leaving home.

MESCALINE (PEYOTE)

Brief History/Social Context

Unless your character's a member of the Native American Church and using peyote for religious ceremonies, he may have a hard time legally buying it in most US states. With hallucinogenic effects similar to LSD (acid), mescaline is contained in parts of certain southwestern cacti, such as the little disc-shaped buttons of *Lophophora williamsii*, better known as the peyote cactus. This cactus has long been used as a naturally occurring source of mescaline in religious ceremonies by indigenous peoples across the Southwest and Mexico. Like other hallucinogens, mescaline is being researched for the treatment of depression and addiction. But growing, buying, selling, and consuming the peyote cactus is heavily regulated and restricted. Until recently, the only legal commerce in the US was in Texas where licensed peyote growers and sellers (peyoteros) have been authorized to sell solely to the Native American Church and must register with the Drug Enforcement Administration (DEA).

Your character might get mescaline by growing his own cactus or buying powdered cactus online.

But if your character can't legally get peyote, he can still get mescaline. Private use of mescaline is popular and predominantly involves the use of other less widely known species of cacti that contain the hallucinogen, such as the San Pedro cactus. These cacti are legal in the US and can be purchased or grown. Cactus cuttings and pre-dried cactus powder from these legal plants can also be purchased online for easier use. Users then have varying ways to obtain the illicit mescaline chemical from the products. In addition, a synthetically made powdered mescaline (mescaline hydrochloride) has become more widely available.

Mescaline can be developed into your story much like other hallucinogens, with the exception that the effects will last much longer and your character will not be able to function in social settings while tripping. In addition, mescaline scenes lend themselves more realistically to quiet, secluded experiences, as opposed to tripping while in a club or at a party.

A mescaline trip isn't a good choice for plotting into a party scene.

Keep a watch on the rapidly changing legal landscape regarding mescaline, also. Currently, at the federal level *all* forms of mescaline remain illegal in the US with the exception of ceremonial peyote. However, since 2019, there has been a growing move within individual states to decriminalize or legalize mescaline. For example, Colorado has legalized the chemical, including the possession, use, and home cultivation of mescaline producing cacti.

If you're planning to develop a ceremonial scene with mescaline, having the character use the natural plant source, not the synthetic powder, would be more appropriate. In addition, getting a critique partner or sensitivity reader who's a member of the Native American Church will be very important to accurately and respectfully portray this culture.

A sensitivity reader is highly recommended for scenes involving the use of ceremonial mescaline.

So, what makes mescaline so popular? It produces hallucinations and is said to create a prolonged happy mood and a deeper sense of empathy for other people and the world. But, like other hallucinogens, it has a dark side. The hallucinations can offer your character deep revealing visions about life or morph into a frightening experience, especially if he's been depressed or suffered recent emotional stresses. He'll have no control over the bad trip, especially if he's inexperienced using mescaline. Without a trip sitter to help guide his thoughts and fears, he can spiral into extreme emotions, scattered and paranoid thoughts, and unsettling visual hallucinations. Later, memories of the bad trip can cause him anxiety attacks.

Emotional stress can turn your character's enjoyable journey into a frightening experience.

Persistent hallucinations can continue long after your character's high is gone.

Although rare, months after using mescaline, your character could also suffer an unnerving flashback—a momentary reliving of a previous trip, either good or bad. Flashbacks can occur spontaneously or be triggered by stressful life events. Another rare phenomenon is called Hallucinogen Persisting Perception Disorder (HPPD). With this condition, your character will continue to experience visual hallucinations and distorted perceptions, such as light trails behind moving objects, intense world colors, or objects that don't exist, even long after a trip ends. HPPD will interfere with his daily life and can continue indefinitely. He may be unable to function normally in society, lose his job, and become severely depressed.

Slang Terms

(Since terminology and slang terms change over time, further research is highly encouraged.)

Street names

big chief, buttons, cactus, mesc, mescal, Pedro, peyote, San Pedro, SP, TDM, Peruvian Torch

Other terms

- Journey: the visual, auditory, and emotional experience from mescaline, as in "My last mescaline journey was intense." Also called trip.
- Tek: short for "technique" and often refers to one of many chemical processes used to extract mescaline from cactus, as in "I have a great tek that gives me a high yield."
- Trip, tripping: the visual, auditory, and emotional experience from mescaline. Also called journey.

Weaving the Plot

How is it used?

Fresh or dried parts of the cactus (such as peyote buttons or cactus stalks) are chewed or made into tea. Some users cook the cactus parts for hours then strain them to separate the drinkable juice from the pulp. Every user has personal preferences for how to do this, from freezing the cactus first to simply chopping it up. Some use Crock-Pots or slow cookers to liquify the pulp, while others use a series of chemical extractions to product crystalized mescaline. Because of the extremely bitter taste, some users prefer to place their ground cactus or synthetic mescaline powder into gel capsules or dilute it in strong flavored juices, such as grapefruit juice. Alternatively, the powders can be smoked.

Now you try it

How will my character act or feel?

During the "come up" of the high, stomach ache, nausea, and vomiting can occur, especially with swallowed mescaline. Your character should keep a vomit bucket and fresh drinking water nearby. He may also decide to have more mescaline within reach in case he wants to take a "bump up" to elevate the high later. Audible buzzing and small visual changes, such as vibrations of objects, walls, and people, will be his first signs his trip is beginning. A mellow happiness and a sudden, deep empathy for others will fill him. Visually, the hallucinations can include objects and people morphing from one shape to another. For example, a chair can develop arms or the walls may begin to melt. As the euphoria increases, depth perception and balance are lost. Colors will appear more vivid and your character will "hear colors" or "see sounds." Walking will become harder, as will judging the distance of objects. Similar to LSD, the high includes a warped sense of time and space. Awareness of the real surroundings can fade in and out. For example, your character may see a tunnel that doesn't exist while simultaneously talking to his friend that actually is present. Frighteningly, users have reported driving cars while tripping, uncertain of how they got to their final destination but remembering hallucinating during the drive.

Your character will hear colors, see sounds, and watch objects morph.

If your character is in a relaxed, quiet place, an enjoyable, calm trip is realistic. But outside sounds, dangers, and influences can quickly turn the trip into a frightening experience. Local gunfire, ambulance sirens, or watching a horror movie can trigger frightening hallucinations, such as monsters attacking or human body parts strewn on the floor. Paranoia and panic can develop—he may fear people are trying to hurt or capture him. He likely won't be able to mentally or physically control his actions or reactions unless he's very experienced with mescaline trips. Without a trip sitter for safety, he may try to get away from these horrifying visions and unwittingly walk into dangers. For example, if your character decides to escape the visions, he could accidentally walk into traffic or off of a ledge he cannot see.

Without a trip sitter, your character could accidentally walk into life-threatening situations.

If the character ends up in the emergency room, agitated, combative, and frightened by his hallucinations, there are no antidotes to stop the trip. The doctors will only be able to sedate him, treat his symptoms, and wait for the mescaline to wear off.

Flashbacks offer unexpected twists. These can occur long after the character's last mescaline experience—from a few days to more than a year. Although flashbacks only last a few seconds to minutes, they can be very unsettling. And if your character doesn't know why he relived those visions, he may believe he was drugged or worry that he's losing his mind.

Hallucinogenic flashbacks can frighten your character and those around him.

If your character chronically uses mescaline, he may develop long-term effects, such as memory and speech difficulty, depression, suicidal thoughts, and psychosis.

Now you try it

> **Writing Prompt #2** Write a scene involving a grandfather whose favorite granddaughter secretly empties his vitamin capsules, refilling them with powdered mescaline. Why does she do this? What happens to her grandfather?

How long will this drug affect my character?

The "come up" can take from thirty minutes to an hour, during which time some hallucinatory effects will slowly increase. It's often said the first hour is a game of patience, the second hour is bliss. The main effects will peak around two to four hours into the trip and can last from eight to twelve hours.

Putting It All Together

> **Sample Scenario** Dylan sips the steaming tea, grimacing with each swallow. Raindrops trickle down the windowpane, the willow sways in the yard. He waits, absorbing the calm. Soon, he leans over the trash can, vomits, and then curls up, willing the nausea to go away. When it finally does, he slowly props himself up and laughs. He loves this part. The walls are shimmering and slowly melting into the carpet. The room's vibrating, sending streaks of energy cresting from one side of the room to the other before disappearing into the wall. Out his window, the raindrops melt the trees into the ground.

Now you try it

> **Writing Prompt #3** Your character is trying his first mescaline trip. Write a scene from the trip sitter's point of view, as a bad experience begins to seep into the trip.

Dextromethorphan/DXM

Brief History/Social Context

Does it surprise you to find a common cough syrup in the hallucinogen chapter? It might surprise you more to learn that dextromethorphan (DXM) is chemically related to codeine and morphine. In fact, in the late 1950s, DXM slowly began to replace codeine to treat coughs. At typical doses for coughs, DXM is generally safe. But higher amounts cause euphoria, visual hallucinations, and out-of-body trips. So, swigging several extra doses of DXM syrup to calm a nasty cough can turn into quite an adventure for your character.

> The common cough medicine DXM is a hallucinogen at high doses.

After access to codeine was restricted to requiring a prescription to curb growing abuse, teens and young adults turned to DXM, finding an inexpensive and readily accessible hallucinogenic high. Since then, the rapid rise in DXM abuse has led to attempts to restrict access to it as well. Check the laws of the setting where your plot is unraveling as the sale of DXM to minors is restricted in many locales. Your scene set in 2020 won't feel genuine if your sixteen-year-old character can easily purchase a couple of bottles of DXM syrup for his party. Like buying alcohol underage, the scene will be more genuine if he uses a fake identification card or coerces an older teen to make the purchase. It's also not uncommon for DXM to be shoplifted.

Between wrong doses, drug and herbal remedy interactions, hallucinations, and the risk of making poor decisions while high, DXM offers a variety of interesting scenarios for authors. For example, a character's poor choice to drive a car while tripping on cough syrup might be the last thing he does. Mixing antidepressants or certain herbal supplements with high doses of DXM can land a character in the intensive care unit, suffering seizures and liver failure. Was your character able to buy DXM powder or tablets on the internet? If so, you may be about to write a nasty plot twist since some internet supplies have been tainted with methamphetamine (see "Methamphetamine" in chapter 15). Need a red herring? Urine drug screens can mistakenly identify DXM as the hallucinogen PCP (phencyclidine), leaving your character with some explaining to do. Who knew a simple cough syrup could lend itself to so many plot variations?

Another unique twist can involve the genetic risk that some people have for accelerated DXM side effects. In this case, a character swigging several extra doses of cough syrup on the way to a board meeting might start feeling pretty high in front of the corporate executives. Want to make it worse? Have him also drink grapefruit juice to ward off that cold. Grapefruit juice slows down the metabolism of DXM, causing a bit more of a high than expected. That board meeting will be *very* interesting.

Slang Terms

(Since terminology and slang terms change over time further research is highly encouraged.)

Street names

dex, DXM, orange crush, poor man's PCP, red devils, robo, roboshots, syrup head, velvet

For combination cold tablets containing DXM: CCC, skittles, Triple C

Other terms

- Dexing: using DXM to get high.
- Polistirex: generically used to refer to an extended-release DXM syrup.

- Robotripping: using DXM to get high. Term comes from the originally abused brand name, Robitussin (see "A Note of Caution: Using Brand Names" in chapter 1).
- Skittling: taking multi-symptom cold tablets (which contain several ingredients including DXM) to get high. The term comes from the abuse of Coricidin HBP, multi-symptom tablets which look similar to colorful candies (see "A Note of Caution: Using Brand Names" in chapter 1).

Weaving the Plot

How is it used?

Dextromethorphan comes as a syrup (regular and twelve-hour extended-release), caplets, chewable tablets, lozenges, and dissolvable strips. Usually, the regular syrup is abused since the extended-release version can cause prolonged trips. Doses much larger than those for coughs are used to get high and hallucinate. Because of the sugary, medicinal taste, your character may add the syrup to a flavored soda to make drinking large amounts more palatable. If your character is familiar with abusing DXM, he might target a specific "plateau" dose (see table 10.1). Plateaus indicate how much DXM is needed to get the desired experience.

> Your character might pour his DXM into soda to mask the taste.

DXM is also available in multi-symptom cold tablets, nicknamed Triple Cs. If your character is taking large quantities of these, his DXM trip will be coupled with all the risks from high doses of the other ingredients in the tablets, including decongestants (stroke, heart attack), antihistamines (hallucinations), and acetaminophen (liver failure). Other drugs, such as alcohol or marijuana, are often used at the same time as DXM, increasing the risk of dangerous effects.

Now you try it

Writing Prompt #1 Write a scene involving a teen character convincing his mom to buy more syrup for his "cough." How does the scene evolve when she looks in the medicine cabinet for the large bottle that she just bought a few days ago only to find none? Is your character sly enough to convince her she's mistaken? (You'll continue this scene in Writing Prompt #2.)

How will my character act or feel?

At normal or even slightly high doses, your character can feel relatively nothing. In fact, this may be his reason for deciding to take much more DXM than he should. How the scene unfolds will depend on just how much DXM your character takes. Once he's taken more than a typical dose, it's realistic for him to experience a relaxed euphoria or a slightly drunk sensation. He may begin to see light sparkles or mild color distortions, even with his eyes closed. At high doses, visual hallucinations and a disconcerting out-of-body experience can occur.

The table below describes the general symptoms associated with DXM as the dose escalates. When building these into a scene, keep in mind that real life experiences won't be as precisely delineated as the table but more of a continuum. So, feel free to use creative license to slightly blur the lines between plateaus. However, don't have higher plateau symptoms, such as zombie-like walking, happen with a low dose, like that used for calming a cough.

An out-of-body experience can occur during your character's DXM high.

Bad trips, including nightmarish visions or panic attacks, can be triggered by tripping on DXM during stressful or depressed situations. What if a stressed-out, overwhelmed mom takes several large doses of DXM to calm her cough, flushing it down with her morning grapefruit juice, before rushing out the door to drive the kids to school? Between her anxiety and mental exhaustion, her "trip" to school might be very sparkly . . . if not dangerous.

Need a page-turner? If that stressed-out mom above already takes antidepressants, when she takes that extra DXM she can develop Serotonin Syndrome with symptoms that can range from mild, such as tremors and diarrhea, to life-threatening, including an extremely high body temperature and seizures. This same scenario works for a character using cocaine or some "antidepressant" herbals together with DXM. More information on this condition can be found using the search term *serotonin syndrome*.

Combining certain herbal remedies or cocaine with DXM can be deadly for your character.

Withdrawal symptoms can occur with chronic DXM abuse, leaving your character suffering from nausea, vomiting, and nightmares.

Table 10.1. DXM Plateau Chart: (Note: different "plateaus" may overlap one another)

Amount of Drug	Character's Behavior (brief overview)
Low dose "First Plateau"	Initially a mild stimulant effect and heightened alertness that gives way to slightly drunk behavior, such as a mild imbalance when walking; light-headed and relaxed euphoria, but able to interact socially; body feels heavy; sounds, such as music, are louder and may sound more beautiful; colorful spots of light or sparkles may be seen in surroundings.
Medium dose "Second Plateau"	"Stoned" or "high" feeling and the start of a more dreamlike state; sociable, but harder to focus and function; stomach may hurt and character may vomit; poor coordination can make the character seem clumsy and he may stagger or fall when walking; his legs will look stiff when walking, like a marionette doll; visual hallucinations occur when the character closes his eyes; he can be portrayed with slurred speech, confusion, and mental fogginess; his vision will be choppy, almost like watching strobe lights or a movie briefly freezing on each frame; a drop in inhibitions may cause him to say things he would normally keep private or speak more honestly, almost like a "truth serum."
High dose "Third Plateau"	Very introspective, not good socially, and prefers being alone; visual, sound, and depth distortions occur (such as extremely loud sounds, the world may swiftly tilt back and forth, or the hallway can look unnaturally long); very delayed reactions.
Higher doses "Fourth Plateau"	"Zombie-like" walking, out-of-body experiences that can be frightening and interpreted as death, interactions with higher powers or alien beings, hallucinations, and delusions; he won't understand what's happening and will feel detached from his body; the character may be completely immobile or wander into physical danger, especially if there is no trip sitter; he won't respond to conversations and may not recognize the people around him; other characters might see his eyes darting back and forth rapidly, if they're open; agitation can turn into panic or paranoia; a dangerous rise in body temperature can lead to a rapid heart rate, seizures, and organ damage; if his breathing becomes dangerously slow (or stops), coma and death may follow.

Now you try it

How long will this drug affect my character?

Effects start in about twenty to thirty minutes but can take an hour. Your character can be high for a couple of hours (with smaller doses) or have hallucinations lasting five to six hours (with higher doses). Did someone accidentally (or purposefully!) give your character a large amount of extended-release DXM? If so, he'll have an unexpectedly long trip of twelve hours or more.

After the DXM high wears off, hangover effects, such as feeling sluggish and the inability to concentrate, can last up to a full day depending on how much DXM was taken. With fourth plateau doses, however, assuming your character isn't in a coma or dead, the hangover can last two days or longer.

PUTTING IT ALL TOGETHER

Sample Scenario #1 Morgan takes a deep swig of cough syrup. It goes down easily. He waits, but after a while, nothing has happened, so he swigs the rest of the bottle. Just as he's opening another bottle of DXM, the room fills with sparkly lights. He reaches up to touch the sparkles, gets dizzy, and staggers to the couch. The entire weight of his body seems to slip away as he stares at the patterns moving on the wall.

Sample Scenario #2 Liam notices Peyton standing in the corner at the party, holding the wall. She's talking, but her words are garbled, as if her tongue is numb. Her eyes are frantic, wide.

"Where are the monsters?" she cries out. She walks a few feet, her legs jerking stiffly, before falling onto a couch, moaning, staring blankly ahead.

Now you try it

11

INHALANTS

Brief History/Social Context

Inhalants work well for scenes involving middle school through middle-aged adult characters looking for a quick high. Inhalants include almost any product releasing intoxicating fumes, such as glues, paints, cleaning fluids, spray paints, gases, solvents, gasoline, aerosol sprays, and many others. To restrict access to these dangerous chemicals, stores often keep these products in locked displays and require a minimum age for purchase. Other inhalants, like whipped cream canisters, whippits (metal gas-filled cartridges inside the whipped cream dispensers), and compressed air spray dusters, are readily available. Paint thinners and gasoline can often be found at home in a garage. The fumes from these products are popular to abuse due to the rapid euphoria and head rush they cause. Certain inhalants are abused during "chemsex" (the use of drugs to enhance sexual encounters) and the practice of sexual asphyxiation. Inhalants tend to be abused more by men than women.

Your character might use anything with an intoxicating fume to get high.

With the quick on-and-off high, easy access, and legal status of these chemicals, inhalants are often mistakenly considered less dangerous than other abused drugs. But what abusers don't realize is the high price paid for those few seconds of euphoria: these chemicals all cause brain-cell destruction, either through a dramatic drop in oxygen or direct chemical brain damage. Inhalants are also extremely addictive—with such a short high, users often take numerous repeated doses to regain the euphoria. And inhalants can be deadly. Sudden Sniffing Death from rapid drops in oxygen, even with the first high, is one of the main causes of death from these chemicals.

A few of the more popularly abused chemicals are discussed below, although there's a plethora of abused inhalants, with new chemicals continually being added to the list.

Poppers

Poppers is the common term for a group of related chemicals known as alkyl nitrites. The most well-known of these is amyl nitrite, which began in the late 1800s as a treatment for angina, a painful heart condition. In the middle of an angina attack, a patient would sniff amyl nitrite vapors, causing blood vessels to quickly dilate and reducing the painful pressure against their heart. But this same mechanism also causes a head rush, as well as an increased sex drive and decreased inhibitions. It didn't take long for these latter effects to turn amyl nitrite from a useful treatment to a major drug of abuse. Today's poppers may be amyl nitrite or any of a long list of chemical cousins that create similar effects.

> Inhalants offer characters a cheap, addictive high while offering authors an endless list of dangerous plot twists.

Your character could become addicted to poppers for the high, but they have also become popular to use in chemsex, sexual asphyxiation, and in the LGBTQ+ community—creating a wide variety of options for plots and character backgrounds.

So, why are they called poppers? Historically, medical amyl nitrite was sold in little glass ampules that made a small popping sound when cracked open. Amyl nitrite and related chemicals are still referred to as poppers, even though many are now packaged in small bottles with screw-off caps. When the lid is unscrewed, the liquid rapidly turns into a vapor to sniff. The bottle must be quickly reclosed to save the rest of the contents from evaporating.

> Don't have your character leave the lid off of his popper or all of the drug will rapidly evaporate.

When amyl nitrite moved to prescription-only status to reduce abuse, its related cousins became readily available (and continue to be sold) in paraphernalia shops, sex shops, and—more recently—online, labeled as "sex enhancer," "liquid aroma," or "video head cleaner."

Glues and solvents

Glues and solvents are popular for their rapid high. Abused glues, such as model airplane glue, typically have strong aromas from various intoxicating solvents. Other solvents include a wide range of strong-smelling chemicals, such as paint thinners, cleaners, and nail polish remover. Felt-tip markers with intoxicating aromas were at one time heavily abused, but many have been redesigned to no longer produce the fumes. Ethyl chloride spray, usually used to temporarily numb the skin before injections and piercings, is increasingly abused. Solvents cause euphoria by dropping brain oxygen levels, which, in turn, causes brain cell damage, making these chemicals very dangerous.

Nitrous oxide (laughing gas)

Nitrous oxide is an anesthetic gas used during some medical, dental, dermatological, and veterinary procedures. It's also used as a foaming agent in whipped cream canisters. (Don't get this drug confused with nitric oxide—an inhaled drug used to help with certain severe lung conditions.) Low nitrous oxide doses can cause mild relaxation and giggling, but high doses create an intense euphoria and a disconnection from the body. Nitrous oxide can work well for younger characters using either whipped cream cannisters or whippits to get high. It's also realistic for your health professional protagonist (such as a dentist), although this character's more likely to get high on the medical nitrous oxide that's available for procedures, such as during a dental extraction.

Slang Terms

(Since terminology and slang terms change over time, further research is highly encouraged.)

Street names

- Amyl nitrite: amys, bold, butt relaxer, climax, jungle juice, liquid gold, liquid incense, poppers, rush, snapper, super rush
- Glues: gluey, snotballs (rubber cement balls lit and the released vapor inhaled)
- Nitrous oxide: laughing gas, whip-it, whippit, hippie crack

Other terms

- Bagging: breathing fumes from a bag.
- Dusting: refers to spraying an aerosol into the mouth or nose; also describes sprinkling the hallucinogen PCP (phencyclidine) onto marijuana.

- Glading: sniffing air freshener.
- Huffing: inhaling fumes through the mouth (from a container or a rag).
- Sniffing: inhaling fumes through the nose.

Weaving the Plot

How is it used?

All inhalant drugs are abused by inhaling fumes in some fashion. No matter the source, it's realistic to have a character take back-to-back doses to try to stay high. He'll carry the whippit cartridge, bottle of glue, or can of air duster with him, taking hit after hit. Uncapped markers and glues are sniffed directly from the container. Some thick glues, like rubber cement, can be balled up and lit on fire, with the fumes inhaled as the glue melts. Most of the liquids can be directly poured into a closable container, like a balloon, with fumes quickly inhaled through the opening. The container must be rapidly closed before the remaining fumes escape. These fumes can also be inhaled (huffed) from paper bags containing chemical-soaked rags or cotton balls. Your character would take repeated huffs from the bag, getting high from his own carbon dioxide as well as the fumes. For poppers, the cap is screwed off, the fumes are quickly inhaled, and the bottle is rapidly resealed. If your story takes place when amyl nitrite was in glass ampules, the character should snap the ampule open (there will be a small popping sound) to inhale the fumes. Or he might dip a cigarette into the liquid and inhale the fumes through the unlit cigarette. Getting small shards of glass in a finger while cracking open the ampule is realistic.

Looking for an explosive danger? Amyl nitrite can combust near a flame. If lit, that amyl nitrite–dipped cigarette could burst into flame, severely burning your character's face and eyebrows. If your readers have been primed to know the danger, they'll be on the edge of their seats, wondering what will happen as the character lights that match.

A lit popper-dipped cigarette will severely burn your character.

Medical nitrous oxide is usually stored in a large tank. During procedures, the gas is blended with oxygen for the patient's safety and then either inhaled from the end of a tube (for some facial skin procedures) or through a small mask over the nose, such as at the dentist. The flow of gas is slowly increased during the procedure to create the right amount of relaxation for the patient. When abused, the gas flow is increased even more to achieve a high. To get a hit (a dose) of nitrous oxide from a whippit, your character can inhale gas directly from a whipped cream can. He must hold the can upright so the cream doesn't escape while he's releasing the gas into his mouth. If he's using just the whippit cartridge (removed from the can), the escaping gas and container become extremely cold—enough to burn his fingers or damage his lungs. To avoid this, he can release the gas into a balloon and allow it to warm up before taking a hit. If your character's been doing this awhile, he may use a "cracker," a device that pops a hole in the whippit canister, allowing the gas to move into a chamber and warm up before being inhaled. This helps reduce the risk of lung damage from breathing in the freezing cold gas and makes an easy redosing dispenser to carry. Images of these products can be found online using the search terms *hippie crack, whippits, and nitrous oxide.*

Now you try it

> **Writing Prompt #1** Choose one of your own characters to have an inhalant addiction. How did this habit begin and why? Which inhalant would this character abuse? (You'll use this information in Writing Prompt #2.)

How will my character act or feel?

Overall, for most of these drugs, your character will feel a rapidly intense head rush and dizziness. Inhibitions will drop and sexual arousal will peak. Drowsiness, difficulty thinking, and slurred speech are all realistic for your character to experience until the high wears off. He may vomit, pass out, or both. Brief hallucinations and sound distortions often occur during the height of the head rush. When the high wears off, your character can continue to have a foggy mind or tiredness for several more minutes to hours. When he meets other characters in a scene, they'll be able to smell an odd chemical odor on his breath and clothing.

Chest pain followed by a heart attack is possible during any inhalant abuse, as are seizures. Sudden Sniffing Death can happen during the character's very first high, as the rapid drop in oxygen shuts down his heart and brain. He could also die from asphyxiation (when "bagging"), choke on vomit while passed out, or have an accident while high (such as crashing a car while huffing).

Sudden Sniffing Death can kill a character the first time he gets high with an inhalant.

For all of these drugs, since the euphoria goes away so quickly, what starts out as a seemingly harmless high will rapidly turn into a serious addiction. Your character will soon take repeated doses to stay high. If he tries to stop his habit, he'll only have mild *physical* withdrawal symptoms, like insomnia. But *psychologically*, his desire for the high will overtake everything in his life. For example, a high school character might be driven to keep getting high, despite plummeting grades, lost college scholarships, getting kicked off the sports team, and failing out of school. This *could* paint an interesting backstory for a character driven to help other teens avoid this fate.

Irreversible effects from chronic inhalant abuse can plague your character, including permanent limb spasms from nerve damage, hearing loss, and permanent disabilities from brain damage (see the appendix).

Surviving a past huffing addiction can paint a compelling backstory for a character.

A few additional details related to specific inhalants are included below to help with plotting.

Poppers. These will give your character a massive dizzying head rush (high), fast heartbeat, flashes of light (similar to seeing stars), a pounding (thumping) headache, face flushing, and possibly a rush of sexual energy. Did he accidentally touch the popper to his nose while sniffing? He should wince at the small, painful chemical skin burns that will later become tell-tale yellow scabs around his nose and lips. He needs to be careful to recap the bottle after he sniffs the vapors to avoid spilling the liquid onto his skin. This can be hard to remember while his head is spinning and his vision is clouded over. If the liquid splashes into his eyes, it will be extremely painful. Flushing his eyes for several minutes with water *might* help save his vision. Or you can believably decide he develops permanent vision loss. Accidentally drinking the popper liquid can cause severe mouth and throat burns along with the risk of a life-threatening condition called methemoglobinemia, where the body can't carry enough oxygen in the blood. This will cause him to develop a light blue-gray or purplish tinge to his lips, skin, and fingernails. And if his blood is drawn in a lab, it will appear chocolate brown in the tube. With methemoglobinemia, the character will have a bad headache, feel exhausted, won't be able to think clearly, and will breathe rapidly, as his body tries to find enough oxygen. This can worsen, with your character passing out, having seizures, slipping into a coma, and dying. An antidote called methylene blue is available if he gets to an emergency room in time. Shortages of methylene blue have occasionally occurred—*there's* another potential twist!

Light blue-gray or purple skin and exhaustion can be the first signs that your character has a life-threatening condition.

Using sildenafil (Viagra) while high on poppers can cause a deadly, sudden drop in blood pressure. Your character will get dizzy, pass out, and without emergency help, die.

Glues and Solvents. These chemicals cause a pounding head rush. Your character may realistically sleep with his bottle to continue taking hits (doses) periodically. Repeated brain damage with regular use can leave permanent disabilities from mild to severe (see the appendix), making everyday tasks difficult.

Nitrous Oxide (laughing gas). Nitrous oxide whippits will make your character act like a "happy drunk" within seconds. He'll feel relaxed, lightheaded, tingling, dizzy, giddy, and will probably be laughing or giggling. The high will go away rapidly (within a few seconds to a minute). When used for medical procedures, your character will also feel lightheaded and giddy, but a deeper high occurs when the gas is abused. With these higher doses, after the initial giggly stage, he can experience an intense loud buzzing sound, with his vision clouding over, similar to white static on a television screen. He won't be able to control his movements and will feel detached from his body and the surroundings. Once he stops breathing the vapors, the effects will fade over a few minutes. A spontaneous abortion or infertility can be faced by a character that's accidentally been exposed to nitrous oxide regularly at work. Special masks are used in some medical facilities so the nitrous oxide does not get into the air to keep the workers, such as dental hygienists, safe from these risks.

Now you try it

> **Writing Prompt #2** Write a scene using the character you developed in Writing Prompt #1. He's getting high with a friend. What does the scene look like? How will the character feel?

How long will this drug affect my character?

Whether sniffed or huffed, these chemical vapors rapidly cross into the brain, creating a high within seconds. The high can last from one to several minutes, depending on the chemical. An exception is when nitrous oxide is used for a medical or dental procedure, since it's given almost continuously, with the dose carefully controlled to achieve the right effects. Any effects from the gas reverse over a few minutes after it's turned off.

PUTTING IT ALL TOGETHER

Sample Scenario #1 Marlow lays back in the chair as the loud buzz of the skin laser starts. She holds a tube to her lips, breathing the white mist coming out of the end.

"Keep breathing that so you don't feel the pain," the technician says. "I turned it up good and high."

Marlow takes a few breaths but turns her head away, giggling. The technician pushes the tube back to her mouth, urging her to take deeper breaths. As she does, a loud buzzing fills Marlow's ears. The room becomes fuzzy, covered in white stars. She can't see the technician. Can't feel her body. She panics, pulling away from the tube, then braces until the room comes back into view. She flinches at the pain of the laser.

"I told you, keep breathing the gas," demands the technician. "I can't have you moving around like that."

Sample Scenario #2 Finley walks into the dark foyer, struggling with the bags in her arms. That's odd, she thinks. Jesse should be home. She stubs her toe on the way into the kitchen before finally placing the bags on the table and reaching for the light. She gasps. Jesse is slumped over a chair, a pile of spray cans at his feet, his eyes glazed over.

Now you try it

Writing Prompt #3 Two teens are driving down the highway. One huffs deeply from a paper bag, closing his eyes as the rush hits his head. He offers the bag to the driver. Explore this scene. Does the driver take a hit? What happens next?

12

LEAFY LEFTOVERS

Unfortunately, I cannot cover every possible useful drug for writers, so throughout this book I have chosen to focus on the most interesting or misunderstood as a representative sample. With herbal drugs this becomes a problem, as there is a giant forest (literally) of them to choose from, each with unique effects. So, I have picked a few that, due to social acceptance, safety misconceptions, interesting effects, or mainstream popularity, *have* to be included in this book. The problem is that, while each of these don't warrant their own chapter, their only commonality is having originated from natural plants (and on some level, having been modified since their discovery). That's a loose association, given that the other chapters discuss drugs that are naturally grouped together or can stand alone. And the resolution of this conundrum brings us to the Leafy Leftovers chapter, which could just as easily be titled "Herbals from Natural Plants That Have Been Modified but Are Otherwise Unrelated."

These leafy leftovers include belladonna, kratom, marijuana, and Spice (K2).

BELLADONNA

Brief History/Social Context

Would you put a drug called "deadly nightshade" into your eyes? Believe it or not, in ancient times, women did just that. Why? One of the alkaloid chemicals in the deadly nightshade (belladonna) plant causes very dilated pupils, creating what was considered a beautiful and seductive look. Unfortunately for those women, regular use of belladonna eyedrops could also lead to permanent blurry vision or even blindness.

Various parts of the belladonna plant have been used for centuries to treat many ailments. Belladonna plasters were historically used to treat everything from muscle aches to colic. Believe it or not, up until the early 1900s, belladonna was even a component of "asthma cigarettes," smoked as treatment during asthmatic attacks. It's also been used in religious ceremonies and abused to cause hallucinations.

The plant remains a popular herbal medicine today to treat a wide range of illnesses, from comforting upset stomachs to use as a sedative. But the dose must be carefully measured since every part of the belladonna plant contains alkaloids that can be poisonous in the wrong dose. For example, adding too many leaves to tea can cause severe poisoning symptoms or even death. And eating just a small handful of the plant's sweet, dark purple berries is fatal. In fact, the plant's formal name, *Atropa belladonna*, combines the Italian word for *beautiful woman* (belladonna) with the name of the Greek fate responsible for ending life (Atropos).

Eating just a small handful of belladonna berries can be lethal for your character.

Belladonna plants contain a group of alkaloid chemicals that have many proven medicinal benefits. Eventually, these alkaloids were extracted from the plant to create safer medicines and leave behind the potentially toxic chemicals. These medicines are widely used today. You may have used one, such as a scopolamine patch to prevent motion sickness or hyoscyamine pills to calm an irritable bowel. Atropine, another alkaloid, may have been used to dilate your pupils or to decrease your respiratory secretions during a surgery. It's also used as an antidote for certain poisonings, but hopefully you haven't experienced that! But even belladonna, itself, is still prescribed in suppositories combined with opium to treat irritable bowel syndrome.

Unfortunately, because belladonna can cause a dreamy high and hallucinations, it has a history of abuse. In the days of those asthma cigarettes, abusers were known to crush the cigarette contents and dilute them into a drink to get high. Today, belladonna is abused by chewing on leaves, making teas, or smoking the crushed dried plants. Another plant that's a cousin to belladonna, with similar alkaloids and history of abuse for hallucinations, is jimson weed (*Datura stramonium*). More information on this plant can be found using the search term *jimson weed poisoning*.

Wondering how to take advantage of belladonna or these other alkaloid drugs to raise the stakes for your protagonist? You may have already read stories using belladonna in the plot. It's believed that in Shakespeare's *Macbeth*, the Scottish defeat of the Dane's unconscious army was aided by belladonna-laced water. In a pivotal scene in *The Hunger Games*, by Suzanne Collins, the

Several authors have used belladonna to create suspenseful plot twists. main characters threaten to commit suicide by eating "nightlock" berries, which bear striking similarities to belladonna. And in *Romeo and Juliet,* many believe the potion that allowed Juliet to fake her own death was made from belladonna.

Of course, real life examples also offer great ideas as well. Emergency room visits and poison center calls for belladonna do occur. Agitated, hallucinating patients have been brought to emergency rooms after smoking unknown amounts of belladonna. In some cases, belladonna berries have been mistaken for wild blueberries, ending in hallucinations and severe agitation. Even a homeopathic teething gel containing belladonna led to cases of breathing problems and seizures in infants, resulting in a warning bulletin by the Food and Drug Administration (FDA) in 2010. And in the 1990s, scopolamine-laced heroin resulted in numerous emergency room visits.

With the ever-growing popularity of natural herbal medicine, there has been an increased interest in homegrown medicinal plants. For the expert home gardener, this might not pose any problems. But for your poorly informed novice, trouble could be brewing. How the danger evolves, of course, is all the fun as an author. Does the protagonist fail to warn a house guest about the dangerous berries growing in the garden? Or is she actually an expert horticulturalist that's growing poisonous plants for her own sinister plot?

The medical drugs extracted from belladonna also offer both helpful treatments and the opportunity to build tension in scenes. For example, taking too many hyoscyamine tablets can leave your character suffering from light sensitivity, blurry vision, dizziness, a very dry mouth, difficulty swallowing, hot, dry flushed skin, and a high body temperature. If that's not miserable enough, your character can also be agitated, confused, staggering, and hallucinating (see "Anticholinergic Toxidrome" in chapter 2).

Slang Terms

(Since terminology and slang terms change over time, further research is highly encouraged.)

Street names

deadly nightshade, devil's herb, naughty man's cherries (the berries)

How is it used?

Historically, ground belladonna leaves and roots were smoked or made into teas, eye drops, poultices, and tinctures. Belladonna is still medically used in combination with opium as a suppository to calm irritable bowels. It's also been found in some homeopathic medicines, such as teething gels, and some herbalists recommend belladonna for various ailments. In a contemporary setting, your character could be found smoking belladonna leaves or drinking tea made with them.

Hyoscyamine is available as pills for irritable bowel syndrome. Scopolamine pills are no longer available, but for storylines taking place prior to the early 2000s they were. Some modern compounding pharmacies continue to make pills that they claim are scopolamine-like. Scopolamine skin patches are often prescribed to avoid seasickness, motion sickness, or to prevent vomiting after surgery. And scopolamine has even been used to spike the drinks of unsuspecting victims, similar to roofies (see "Flunitrazepam" in chapter 9). Atropine is used as eyedrops to dilate eyes for procedures, as an antidote for organophosphate poisoning, and to prevent a drop in heart rate that can occur in certain medical situations.

Now you try it

> **Writing Prompt #1** Have some fun developing a scene where one of your own characters, an inexperienced camper, decides to forage for leaves to make into an herbal tea while the other campers pitch their tents. (You'll continue this scene in Writing Prompt #2.)

How will my character act or feel?

Drinking tea or smoking cigarettes made with belladonna or these related alkaloids can cause drowsiness and relaxation. It can also cause an extremely dry mouth, difficulty swallowing, blurry vision, and dilated eyes that are sensitive to light. If your character drinks enough tea, she might be staggering, talking nonsense, and acting very confused. Her heart will be racing and her skin flushed and hot. But don't have her sweating since belladonna blocks this body cooling method. If you want to create more trouble for your protagonist, she can become agitated, have hallucinations, and even become delirious. For example, she can become very upset when she sees imaginary insects crawling all over her kitchen. Or she can wander outside of the house in her delirious state. What happens to her then? Probably something she'll regret, but hopefully something that will grow her character arc. If she just stays home drinking more of her tea, however, she could collapse from a seizure, with foam dripping from her mouth, or fall into a coma. Emergency help will be needed, since her breathing might slow to the point of death.

If your character's using belladonna eyedrops, in addition to those very dilated, seductive eyes, her vision will be blurry and her eyes sensitive to light.

Smoking belladonna can make your character hallucinate.

Not into plant plots? Consider scopolamine patches for some milder belladonna-like symptoms to add trouble to your character's day. Some people are very sensitive to scopolamine patches. If your character doesn't realize she's sensitive to them and uses a couple of patches before going on her evening dinner cruise, she might get more than she bargained for. It takes a few hours for those patch to really work, though, so she'll already be on the cruise and sipping champagne to quench her very dry mouth, when the patches finally take effect. She might seem a bit tipsy to the other cruisers as she slurs her words and staggers around deck. Instead of a fun evening, she might be found dozing on a deck chair. The patches won't be lethal, though, so don't plan on killing this character off.

Interestingly, after a scopolamine patch is removed, some people have an unexpected reaction similar to severe motion sickness that can start a day or two later. So, even after that cruise is done, your poor character can suffer a couple of days of dizziness, headache, nausea, and vomiting.

Now you try it

> **Writing Prompt #2** Continue the scene from Writing Prompt #1. Of course, the leaves your camper found to make the tea fell from a belladonna plant. What happens when all the campers join together sipping the tea by the campfire to keep warm?

How long will this drug affect my character?

Pupil dilation and blurry vision from belladonna eyedrops will occur over an hour and can last from several hours to more than a day. With scopolamine patches, the impact on motion sickness can take about three to four hours. Dry mouth can start much sooner, however. If too many patches are used, your character will also become drowsy, sluggish, and not be able to think clearly. She may seem slightly drunk. And if she touched the patches before rubbing her eyes, within a few minutes her vision will be blurry. Some effects, like mild drowsiness, can continue for several hours after a patch has been removed. But twenty-four to forty-eight hours later, unexpected seasickness-like symptoms can begin and last several days. With hyoscyamine tablets, it can take about an hour for symptoms to begin. The hallucinations and agitation from belladonna tea or berries can begin in less than an hour and last several more. The poison from berries can take five to ten minutes to absorb. If enough berries are eaten, death can quickly follow (within about thirty to sixty minutes).

PUTTING IT ALL TOGETHER

Sample Scenario What a lovely breakfast in bed. Of course, she *deserves* it. If Alex *really* loved her, he'd do this all the time. But the coffee is perfect for a change, the eggs delightful—not watery like he *usually* makes them. She slathers another piece of toast with the delicious dark-purple jam. She's never tasted a jam quite like it. Still, strawberry would be better—it never leaves her mouth this dry. But he never remembers what she likes. She washes the toast down with more coffee and watches a hummingbird fluttering outside her window. After another bite of toast, she blinks and rubs her eyes. Why's everything so blurry. "Alex?" She struggles to swallow her mouthful. "Alex!"

Alex slowly walks in, his blurry figure pausing at the foot of the bed.

"Where have you been? I've been calling you. I don't feel good." The room is spinning. Her hand presses against the thudding in her chest. "What's happening?"

Alex smiles.

She frowns. "Don't just stand there." She fights to keep her eyes from closing. "Help me!" The cup slips from her fingers. "Alex?" she mumbles.

The room grows dark.

Now you try it

Writing Prompt #3 Write a scene where a character is found in the park yelling nonsense and attacking people. His hands and lips are stained purple. The police find his pockets filled with belladonna berries. What happens? Did he only eat a few berries? Or is he in worse trouble? Does he tell the police where he got the berries, before he passes out?

KRATOM

Brief History/Social Context

Need an herbal remedy that can easily add a twist to your plot? Kratom may be a good choice. The kratom plant (*Mitragyna speciosa*) comes from Southeast Asia, where the leaves have been used for centuries to decrease fatigue and treat a variety of ailments, including pain. Different kratom strains are identified by the color of the veins in the leaves: red, green, or white. The effects of kratom can be different, depending on the strain and the dose. Low doses will act like a stimulant for your character, increasing energy, and sociability, while higher doses may help calm her pain or decrease opioid withdrawal symptoms. Or, *she* may use it for other ailments, such as insomnia or anxiety.

Does kratom work? A few small studies show some promise, but there's unfortunately no good information yet supporting its use. Nevertheless, self-treatment using kratom increased after the opioid crisis was declared in 2017, resulting in tight restrictions on prescribing pain pills and leaving many patients to seek other remedies. Since then, its use for quelling withdrawal and anxiety symptoms has also grown.

Your character might start using kratom to self-treat pain or opioid withdrawal.

Even before its recent accelerated use in the US, kratom sparked controversy. Because of safety concerns and potentially dangerous side effects, in 2016 the Food and Drug Administration (FDA) proposed banning kratom. Wide-spread backlash and demonstrations caused the FDA to reverse its recommendation. However, since kratom is unregulated, concerns about product variation and safety led the FDA to warn the public against its use and confiscate shipments coming into the US. Depending on the setting of your story, the regulations related to kratom use will vary. Some states have made kratom illegal to sell or have developed restrictions against sales to minors. Others are creating regulations for safer labeling.

Where will your character get kratom? In states where it's legal, it can be purchased from a variety of stores, such as smoke shops, herbal dispensaries, liquor stores, and even online.

Because kratom is a natural plant, it's often seen as "safe," but it can have some nasty side effects. In high doses, it not only causes euphoria but also nausea, vomiting, agitation, anxiety, tremors (like shaking hands), a rapid heartbeat, and hallucinations. Taking an opioid together with a high dose of kratom can cause breathing to slow to the point of death. Kratom also causes tolerance (where higher doses are needed for the same effect), addiction, and withdrawal.

Characters can suffer hallucinations, addiction, or withdrawal with kratom.

Since kratom isn't regulated, there are no standards for concentration, purity, or quality. The potency of kratom varies widely, depending on how the plants are harvested and dried. And there are fluctuations in the content of kratom capsules, making doses inconsistent. The lack of purity standards has even resulted in contaminated batches causing salmonella poisoning and death.

As an author, you have a lot of freedom to decide not only how and why your character uses kratom but also to plot the kind of trouble she gets into using it. Your young adult may simply use it to soften the anxiety and insomnia suffered while weaning off of a chronic marijuana habit. Or you can weave a more complicated character arc, starting with a grandmother who begins using kratom for her painful arthritis when she's unable to get more opioid pills from her doctor. She could wind up in the hospital, severely ill with salmonella poisoning. Or she might run out of kratom after it becomes illegal in her state. Then, not only could she suffer kratom withdrawal, but her pain will return. This could believably drive your character to seek out street opioids, such as oxycodone. From there, you have many plotting options where her struggles can go from bad to worse. She could become addicted to oxycodone or, when that's no longer enough, move on to heroin or fentanyl (see "Oxycodone," "Heroin," and "Fentanyl" in chapter 13).

Slang Terms

(Since terminology and slang terms change over time, further research is highly encouraged.)

Street names

biak, kakuam, ketum, thang, thom

Other terms

- Green-veined: kratom leaves with green veins and associated with euphoria, as in "I switched to green-veined after the white stopped working."
- Red-veined: kratom leaves with red veins
- White-veined: kratom leaves with white veins

Weaving the Plot

How is it used?

Kratom comes in capsules, extracts, dried leaves, and ground powder. The leaves and powder are extremely bitter and foul tasting. Because of this, kratom is often blended into strong flavored teas, orange juice, smoothies, or peanut butter to mask the taste. One popular method to minimize the taste is called "toss and wash," where the powder is tossed into the user's mouth, quickly followed by a drink, like a flavored sports drink, to flush the dose down. The leaves are also smoked or chewed. Your character may have to rotate various strains or take a drug "holiday" (a few days or longer without doses) to reduce tolerance.

Now you try it

> **Writing Prompt #1** Develop the backstory to one of your own characters that uses kratom. Why does the character use it? What difficulties are faced in getting supplies? (You'll use this background in Writing Prompt #2.)

How will my character act or feel?

Your character's mouth will feel numb after drinking kratom tea or chewing the leaves. With low doses, the character can be portrayed as having a relaxed alertness (like having strong coffee, but without the jitteriness), a more focused mind, and an improved mood. With higher doses, she might feel a buzzy high, drowsiness, and her pain can subside. Because of the high, lightheadedness can make it difficult to walk or think clearly for a short time. If she's been using kratom for a while, it's realistic that she would no longer get any euphoria at all. This may be frustrating, especially if she's specifically using it for the high. She'll have to either keep escalating her doses or take a drug holiday, possibly suffering withdrawal, to undo her tolerance to kratom.

If your character is experiencing withdrawal, she can be yawning, anxious, agitated, have painful muscle aches and spasms, and suffer insomnia. While kratom withdrawal isn't lethal, chronic users say it can be a miserable experience, making it difficult to stop the habit, unless the doses are reduced very slowly over several weeks or more.

Don't have your character die from kratom withdrawal.

Want your character to have a bad experience with kratom? The lingering bitter taste can be strong enough to cause severe nausea. Need it to get worse? If she takes kratom on a full stomach, she's more likely to vomit after the dose. Some people have vomited so much they've ended up in the emergency room, dehydrated and miserably heaving, even once their stomach is empty. *Still* want worse? Your poor character can hallucinate or have a seizure. Kratom can even cause her heart to race, possibly triggering a heart attack, especially if she already has heart problems.

Kratom can send your character to the emergency room with severe vomiting or even a heart attack.

Now you try it

> **Writing Prompt #2** Develop a scene where the character from Writing Prompt #1 has been needing higher doses of kratom recently and is now out of town on a business trip. The airlines lost all the character's luggage, though, which contained all the kratom. What will your character do now?

How long does this drug affect my character?

Within a few minutes of swallowing the tea or chewing the leaves, your character's mouth and throat will feel numb. (If she's a chronic user, this may not happen.) It takes about fifteen to twenty minutes for effects to start—whether euphoria, sedation, or pain relief—and they can last three to four hours.

Sample Scenario She watched the leaves boil in the pot, then strained the brownish liquid into her mug. Grimacing at the bitter taste, she forced herself to quickly gulp the rest. Her stomach heaved, but she swallowed hard, willing her stomach to stay calm. By the time the pot was washed, her tongue was already tingly and numb. Stretching out on the couch, she welcomed the buzzy relaxation and the disappearing ache in her joints.

Now you try it

Writing Prompt #3 Continue your scene from Writing Prompt #2. The luggage is still missing, and it turns out that your character has landed in a state where kratom isn't legal. Withdrawal symptoms are beginning to become uncomfortable. Now what?

MARIJUANA

Brief History/Social Context

As an author, few drugs will be as versatile as marijuana (weed) for making a scene or characters seem realistic. With this natural drug increasingly accepted in society, it'll resonate with a broader base of readers than harder drugs, like heroin. For some of today's adult readers, memories may be triggered of their youth, like sneaking joints behind the school gym. Your character can be anything, from a pot-smoking hippie of the 1960s to a modern-day dabbing college athlete. He can be an adult sneaking his son's pot to get high, a grandpa using medical marijuana for his arthritis, or a teen vaping THC on the way home from school.

Marijuana fits into a wide variety of scene settings and a broad cast of characters.

THC (tetrahydrocannabinol) causes the popular high from marijuana. It comes from the stems, flowers, and leaves of the *Cannabis* plant, which can be dried and then smoked or baked into foods. *Cannabis* extracts are also made into concentrated products, such as hash oil, resin, and wax. These concentrates have up to four times the THC potency of the marijuana plant. With these higher potency products, you can choose to have your protagonist experience a typical marijuana high or increase his troubles with hallucinations and paranoid delusions that seem real and leave him frightened.

Cannabis has increasingly been the focus of many scientific studies for the possible treatment of a wide variety of conditions, such pain or seizures. And although the Food and Drug Administration (FDA) has not formally approved marijuana as a treatment, medical marijuana has been available for several years in a number of US states. However, medical marijuana is not FDA-regulated, so product content and potency vary. The legalization of *recreational* marijuana, available in an increasing number of states, blurs the lines between the different marijuana uses, the kinds of products used, and the laws related to accessing and growing products. With the potency of medical and recreational marijuana almost identical in many cases the distinction between the two products is even further blurred.

Your challenge, as an author, will be to accurately research the legal status of *Cannabis* during the historical setting of your story. A neighborhood shop filled with jars of medical *Cannabis* and THC gummies is believable in many (but not all) states in a contemporary story set in 2020, but not a 1960s historical fiction. For legal information, one resource is the Department of Health for individual states. For a broader look, an online image search using the key phrase *marijuana legalization timeline* offers graphs and charts with information to develop accurate scenarios.

What about understanding trends in marijuana usage? This is one of the drugs that's so commonly used, legally or otherwise, that generations of users exist, each with different slang, devices, and popular strains of weed. An entire industry (both legal and illicit) has developed around growing, selling, and consuming various forms of *Cannabis*, including edibles and smokables. For example, the vaping industry has created a large assortment of products, with special flavors and differing characteristics of the high.

This chapter will help you frame the information in a believable scene, but you should consider doing some good old-fashioned research. Consider interviewing people that used marijuana during the historical time period of your story. Or speak with teens and young adults, who often understand the related language and habits even if they don't use weed themselves. And, if they're legal in your state, you may want to consider visiting a *Cannabis* retail shop (bud or flower shop, "dispensary"), which can give you a wealth of information, making it easier for you to create an accurate

A trip to a *Cannabis* dispensary can help authors more accurately portray modern marijuana use.

and relatable scene. It would also be important to determine any age restrictions for the purchase of recreational marijuana in your setting as it's often restricted to those at least twenty-one years old. This will be the difference between your character making his own purchase in a dispensary or standing outside the shop to beg an adult to buy it for him.

Finally, like many other drugs, street *Cannabis* supplies are increasingly tainted with fentanyl and other illicit drugs, providing potentially deadly twists. Your character may realistically overdose on fentanyl just from smoking marijuana. While the market for "street" weed is declining in states where marijuana is legal, this dangerous scenario could be possible for a character who can't legally buy recreational marijuana and turns to a dealer.

Don't have a character get high from CBD gummies.

CBD is another *Cannabis* chemical. However, the CBD in supplements and skin products is extracted from plants with very little THC. So, don't depict your character getting high from (or addicted to) CBD gummies, although selling homemade CBD lotions could give a character an interesting dimension.

Slang Terms

(Since terminology and slang terms change over time further research is highly encouraged.)

Street names

- Marijuana: bud, devil's lettuce, devil's weed, dope, flower, ganja, grass, greens, herb, Jane, loco weed, Mary Jane, pot, reefer, shit, skunk, trees, weed
- Marijuana concentrates: 710 ("oil" flipped and spelled backward), budder, butane, ear wax, hash, hash oil, honey butter, shatter dabs (dabbing), black oil

Other terms

- Baked (faded, gone, fried, stoned): the feeling of being high on marijuana, as in "He was baked last night."
- Banger: a device used to hold THC concentrate to superheat for dabbing.
- Blunt: a general term referring to marijuana rolled into cigarette papers, as in "Let me hit that blunt."
- Cotton mouth: the feeling of a very dry mouth, as if filled with cotton balls, after using marijuana.

- Cross faded: the extreme high from using alcohol and marijuana together. It often includes severe dizziness, seeing the room spin (worse with closed eyes), disorientation, and panic attacks. As in "Dude, I was so cross faded last night."
- Dabbing: specifically smoking THC concentrates through a device that vaporizes it to inhale, leading to a potent and rapid high; sometimes used generically to mean smoking concentrates in other ways, like vape pens. The popular dance move "dabbing" mimics the teary eyes and forceful cough from inhaling superheated vapor from certain devices: the user quickly turns their face and coughs into the elbow area.
- Dank: high-quality weed, as in "That was some dank shit."
- Delta-8: a legal chemical derived from hemp plants, causes effects similar to, but possibly less potent than, delta-9 THC. In states where marijuana is still illegal, delta-8 sales have increased.
- Delta-9: the main chemical in marijuana that causes the high.
- Dime bag: $10 worth of weed.
- Doobie, joint: a rolled marijuana cigarette (usually in cigarette paper).
- Dub/Dub sack: $20 worth of weed.
- Edibles: food containing marijuana, classically brownies or gummies.
- Faded: slang for very high, as in "I got so faded last night."
- Hit: generally, a single puff (dose) from any device, as in "Let me take a hit off of that." The term is not exclusive to marijuana.
- Hot boxing: involves multiple people smoking weed in a small enclosed area (such as a small car or bathroom) and causing the area to fill with smoke. Inhaling the circulating smoke further intensifies the high.
- Munchies: strong food cravings; marijuana increases appetite, often triggering increased eating while high.
- One-hitter: small, pen-like device holding one single hit of marijuana.
- Pen: various devices for smoking *Cannabis* products in more convenient and less conspicuous ways. May look like a pen, flash drive, or similar object. Examples: vape pen (to smoke vaporized THC concentrates), wax pen (to smoke wax); also "weed pen."
- Ripped: very high.
- Roach: the small, unsmoked portion of a marijuana cigarette. Often salvaged later to smoke and held by a paperclip or clamp.

Sometimes roaches are swallowed to use up the last bits of marijuana.

- Roach clip: a small instrument to hold a roach, like a paper clip or tweezers. Helps avoid burning fingers while holding and passing a lit roach.
- Shake weed: the leftover weed at the bottom of a bag.
- Shatter: a solidified *Cannabis* oil concentrate that has a glass-like appearance.
- Toke: to take a hit of marijuana, often from a rolled cigarette.

Weaving the Plot

How is it used?

Getting medical marijuana requires a special card issued by a physician in many states, although this legal requirement is changing. Dispensaries carry a large assortment of *Cannabis,* with a wide array of names, aromas, and unique characteristics for the experience. These may be dispensed in the natural herb form or as edibles, such as gummies. Recreational marijuana is also sold in dispensaries, in states where it's legal. In states where it isn't, your character can find weed the same way it's been found for decades: through friends, sometimes from parents, growing it, or, notoriously, from dealers. One modern twist is the use of social media apps to buy illicit drugs through a complex system of emojis and slang that has been developed.

There are countless ways marijuana has been used throughout history. The wide range of products (smoked and edible) and the various characteristics of different highs are mind-boggling. For authors, simple and direct marijuana scenes will come across more believable than attempting trendy terminology, specifying weed strains, and laboriously describing how it's used. But in general, when your protagonist buys a bag of recreational *street* weed, after discarding any twigs or stems, the remaining dried leaves and buds of the plant can be rolled in smoking paper, placed into a smoking device (bongs, pipes), baked into foods ("edibles"), or steeped into teas. A supply purchased from a dispensary, however, is often already cleaned of the twigs and stems. If the character is smoking hash oil, wax, resins, or other concentrated THC products he might use a pipe or, for a more contemporary setting, an electronic cigarette or vaping device. Marijuana is used at all times of the day, but "wake and bake" (getting high first thing in the morning) has become popular, especially for regular marijuana users.

Smoking marijuana can leave a distinguishable pungent smell in the air (musky, woody, sweet, or skunky), although this varies by the marijuana strain, the device used, and added flavors. Vaping or dabbing can leave much less odor that dissipates quickly, but a blunt will leave a strong, lingering smell. The odor from using a one-hitter can quickly dissipate because of the small dose size.

Where weed is used has also greatly changed. Before it was widely accepted, smoking weed was generally kept hidden to avoid authority figures. However, the lingering smell of weed in the air or on clothing would be a telltale sign, depending on how it was smoked. So, your teen character, whose mom got a nose-full of a skunky odor when she opened his laundry basket, may have had some explaining to do.

In recent years, it's not uncommon to smell a distinctive marijuana aroma when walking through cities and shopping areas from the public smoking of weed, especially in states where the recreational products are legal. But even in those states, there's a clear delineation of where marijuana smoking is not allowed. For example, it remains illegal to drive while under the influence of marijuana. So, if your character is smoking weed on his way to work, he's as likely to be arrested in 2020 as he would have been in 1980. And smoking or vaping *Cannabis* products can be banned on private properties, like hotels.

> **Smoking marijuana can leave a distinctive odor in the air or on your character's clothes.**

Now you try it

> **Writing Prompt #1** Decide which of your own characters uses marijuana. When did this habit begin and why? How often does the character use it? Would the marijuana be more likely to be smoked or eaten? (You'll use this information in Writing Prompt #2.)

How will my character act or feel?

The magnitude of the effects can be related to the dose and potency of the product. A hit or two of strong weed can bring your character a light euphoria, a feeling of happiness, and some intensified food tastes, yet he can remain sociable. Smoking an entire blunt, however, will bring a more intense high, where the world slows down, stressors are unimportant, and he'll laugh for no reason. His decision-making and reflexes will also become very slow. He won't be able to stay focused on a conversation, pausing mid-sentence and forgetting to continue the thought. And he'll eat, even if he's full ("the munchies"). Some users even become paranoid (such as believing the police are following them), although veteran users can often overcome this fear.

This can offer some fun scene options involving your character's first experience smoking a blunt. Your character may also make bad choices, such as driving a car, while high on marijuana as users are often unaware of their true level of impairment.

Want your character to hallucinate? Smoking potent marijuana strains or THC concentrates can cause hallucinations. They can also realistically occur if your protagonist gets a very high dose of marijuana, such as from consuming too many marijuana edibles. The euphoria from these edibles, such as brownies, can be delayed until digestion occurs. Your character, unaware of this delay, can realistically experience a very intense high and hallucinations after eating several extra brownies before the high begins.

Your character can hallucinate from potent Cannabis.

For chronic marijuana users, withdrawal symptoms can occur, including agitation, sweating, insomnia, and a loss of appetite. Learning and memory impairments can be caused by regular marijuana use as a teen and can offer a backstory for a disability in your adult character.

Now you try it

> **Writing Prompt #2** Using the information from Writing Prompt #1, write a scene depicting the character using marijuana and how it feels. How does the character act?

How long will this drug affect my character?

With smoking and vaping, the high can be felt within a few minutes. Dabbing's effects are rapid (less than a minute). The high can last three to four hours (or longer with more potent products). Eating marijuana-laced foods delays the high for about thirty minutes, due to food absorption, and causes an extended high over several hours, as the marijuana continues to be digested.

PUTTING IT ALL TOGETHER

> **Sample Scenario #1** Arya coughed out a large plume of smoke, signaling Vance to take the pipe. "Dude, I'm so faded right now," he laughed.
>
> Vance took another hit and smiled. "Yeah. That shit's dank!"
>
> Arya stood at the pantry, eating chips out of a bag. "I could use a pizza right now."

Sample Scenario #2 Sam joined the other girls in the kitchen, grabbing another brownie.

"Hey," Carmen said, "put that down! You've already had two."

"But I don't feel anything," Sam complained.

"Oh, you will," Carmen laughed, putting the brownie back. "Give it a few."

Now you try it

Writing Prompt #3 Continue the scene with Arya and Vance (above), as they decide to go get that pizza. What happens as they drive? Do they get lost? Have an accident? How does this scene end?

SPICE/K2

Spice is neither a natural botanical drug nor extracted from leaves. It's a chemical (or several) sprayed onto almost any chopped-up leafy material and then used to get high. Because Spice is thought of as "legal marijuana," it oddly belongs in this chapter. Because it offers great dangerous plot twists, it obviously belongs in this book.

Brief History/Social Context

Need a drug your character would be willing to try, thinking it's safe, but that sends him to the emergency room in a severe panic attack or worse? Starting in 2008, before many states began legalizing marijuana, Spice became a popular legal way to get a marijuana-like high. The euphoria from marijuana is caused by natural cannabinoids. But Spice was made by spraying *synthetic* cannabinoid chemicals onto plant material to smoke or make into tea. Since the original chemicals used were not illegal, and Spice was sold in neighborhood gas stations or smoke shops, it was misinterpreted as safe, making it tempting to people who otherwise might not use a drug. These chemicals also avoided detection on drug screens, further increasing their popularity as a marijuana alternative. The synthetic cannabinoids, however, were *nothing* like the real cannabinoids in marijuana and caused a much more intense, powerful high.

A teen character might smoke Spice to avoid failing a marijuana drug screen but end up with a unexpectedly intense high.

As laws changed making the chemicals in Spice illegal, manufacturers switched to using formulas with a variety of different legal chemicals. The original Spice gave way to increasingly dangerous products, generically now referred to as Spice or K2. With these newer drugs, your character can suffer severe panic attacks, paranoia, hallucinations, or seizures, even during his first high.

Online chat threads about the dangers of Spice, with catchy brand names like Diablo, Brain Freeze, and Mad Hatter, are rampant. The dangers are magnified by the ease of purchasing Spice. Your character will find it in smoke shops, drug paraphernalia stores ("head shops"), and online, sold as "herbal incense" or "potpourri" in colorful pouches or small liquid bottles labeled "not for human consumption" to evade legal restrictions. Ads will lure him, with promises of how great these legal "engineered cannabinoids" can make him feel. Of course, they won't mention that Spice is incredibly addictive. As the cravings consume your character, getting high every day on Spice can cost him his job, his family, and his home.

Spice can send your character to the ER with a panic attack or seizures.

There are also other hidden dangers with Spice. Without manufacturing regulations, users rarely know what they're actually buying. Some packages have no Spice at all, just a variety of chemicals with unknown effects. Poor manufacturing practices have also led to batch contamination. In 2018, over two hundred cases of severe bleeding (hemorrhages) occurred from Spice contaminated with brodifacoum, a blood thinner in rat poison. Emergency rooms reported more cases as recently as 2021. Other batches have been tainted with the deadly opioid fentanyl (*see* Fentanyl in chapter 13). As you can see, your character can get into quite a bit of trouble, if he chooses to use this "safer" alternative to marijuana.

Slang Terms

(Since terminology and slang terms change over time, further research is highly encouraged.)

Street names

bliss, black mamba, blaze, crazy clown, dawn, fake bake, fire, legal weed, no more Mr. Nice Guy, paradise, scooby, sence

How is it used?

Spice/K2 is usually smoked using a pipe, bong, or rolled in cigarette paper, but can also be made into tea. Vaping liquid Spice is becoming increasingly popular. Spice is also sold as a concentrated liquid to drop onto cigarettes (marijuana or tobacco) or to create your own drug-coated rolling papers. Gummies and other edibles made with Spice offer nonsmoking alternatives.

Now you try it

> **Writing Prompt #1** Create a scene where a teenager, who normally wouldn't use drugs, is convinced to vape Spice. Why does the character agree to try it? (You'll continue this scene in Writing Prompt #2.)

How will my character act or feel?

Authors have a lot of freedom to develop scenes since so many different chemicals are sold as Spice. And the "plant material" used can be almost anything, including leaves from dangerous or toxic plants.

A character smoking the original version of Spice can realistically have a high similar to, but more intense than, marijuana, including a pleasant euphoria, giggling, relaxation, difficulty concentrating, drowsiness, and a desire to eat food ("having the munchies"). Or he could experience what's called a "dirty high," feeling as if his "brain is melting" or that he's dying, and then be left with a sickening feeling.

Modern Spice/K2 can give your character a wide range of experiences since the products can have a variety of chemicals with unexpected effects. The drug can leave him feeling intensely high—extremely euphoric, unable to hold a conversation, very drowsy, seeing a dreamy world in slow motion, and unable to function. His heart can feel like it's racing. Or he can have much worse reactions, including a severe panic attack, tremors (shaking as if he's had too much caffeine), agitation, hallucinations, or paranoia. As the high wears off, he'll feel disconnected—unable to tell if he's waking into the real world or still dreaming. Has your character passed out? When he wakes, he might be so disoriented that he panics, becoming combative with anyone nearby.

Your character can have a "dirty high" with Spice, feeling like his brain is melting.

Long after the high has worn off, frightening visions or disturbing thoughts that occurred during the hallucinations can continue to plague your character. For example, some users say they continue to wake up at night, years later, remembering horrifying thoughts or visions that seemed real during the high. Sadly, some users say that using Spice horribly ruined their lives. Others downplay the stories of bad experiences, saying they never suffered these effects.

Frightening visions from a previous hallucination can haunt your character even years later.

Your character can realistically wake in the hospital, after having seizures, even during his first high on Spice. His throat will be too sore to talk when his worried friends gather at his bedside. A nurse can explain that the soreness is from the tube that had to be put down his throat so he could breathe during the seizures. He'll struggle to tell his friends that he can't remember anything after his first couple of hits (doses) of Spice, when his world melted into a terrible dream. That's when he learns that he jumped from the moving car and ran down the road screaming. By the time his friends found him, he was on the ground unconscious, his whole body jerking and foam dripping from his mouth.

If you've decided the character gets Spice tainted with blood-thinner, his first symptoms could be soreness in his low back and side. His urine may be tinged pink or his gums might trickle blood as he brushes or flosses his teeth. These are all signs that a dangerous bleed could be brewing inside him. If you've built the scene tension, your readers will worry when the character ignores these signs and climbs into bed for the night, hoping his high will finally calm down by morning. But when he starts vomiting blood in the middle of the night, he'll realize something is very wrong. With enough internal bleeding, he'll become weak, pass out, and ultimately hemorrhage to death unless he gets emergency medical help.

Now you try it

Writing Prompt #2 Continue the scene from Writing Prompt #1 using your character's point of view during the high. Is it a good experience or does it morph into a terrifying one? End the scene with a page-turner.

How long will this drug affect my character?

Smoking synthetic cannabis causes a high within a few minutes. The high from edibles, such as gummies, will take a little longer to feel due to digestion. Spice tea will take effect in about fifteen minutes. Don't worry about being too specific regarding how long the high lasts since so many different chemicals can actually be in Spice. Consider developing a high lasting from a few to several hours, whichever works for your scene. For Spice contaminated with blood-thinner, let the high wear off, but have the bleeding continue, or worsen, until the character either passes out (and possibly dies) from blood loss or gets emergency medical help. For Spice tainted with other drugs, refer to the individual chapters for ketamine, methamphetamine, or fentanyl for a few ideas. However, choosing a twist with one of these other drugs may cause a more permanent end for your character. For example, a high with fentanyl-laced Spice is likely to be lethal.

PUTTING IT ALL TOGETHER

Sample Scenario #1 Kasey's eyes flutter open. He clenches his teeth at the pounding in his head. A machine beeps loudly next to him. When Kacey looks up at the doctor leaning over him, he sees his smile disappear as his skin turns red and fangs grow from his mouth. Kasey knocks the demon away and scrambles out of the bed. Then the room sways and he crashes to the floor.

Sample Scenario #2 Taylor reaches for the pipe for another hit, but Lee pulls it away.
  "Dude," Lee laughs, "you're so faded right now."
  "Bro," Taylor snorts, "no I'm not." He tries to stop laughing. "Give it!" He grabs the pipe. He fumbles with the lighter and inhales deeply before blowing out another plume of smoke. He tries to stand, but falls back onto the couch, laughing. Then he leans forward, grabbing his chest. His heart is racing, his hands shaking.

Now you try it

Writing Prompt #3 Explore a scene where a character is having frightening hallucinations on Spice and hears a key in the lock of the apartment door. The character reaches for a gun, petrified, just as a friend opens the door. What happens?

13

OPIOIDS

Planning a scene involving a pain pill overdose? Or a rock star shooting up heroin? Want to know if a poppy seed bagel can *really* make your character fail a drug test?

This is your chapter.

With an amazingly long list of opioids, this chapter focuses on some of the most well-known drugs and their key differences useful in developing unique scenes. The dangerous street opioids, such as fentanyl, that are causing an ongoing surge in overdoses and deaths are also highlighted.

CODEINE

Brief History/Social Context

Known on the street as "Captain Cody," codeine is made from opium and has been used medically since the mid-1900s. It's usually combined with promethazine (an antihistamine) in cough syrup or with acetaminophen in tablets (called T3's or T4's) to treat pain. Unfortunately, codeine causes an addictive high and can lead to potentially lethal overdoses. It's considered a "gateway drug"—codeine abusers move on to other opioids, like oxycodone or heroin, seeking a better high.

Codeine pills have long been abused. But abuse of codeine syrup first became popular during the 1960s blues music scene in Texas with a drink called "Lean," "Purple," or "Syrup." This drink combines soda with an opiate cough syrup, such as codeine-promethazine syrup. A hard, fruit-flavored candy is usually added to mask the potency and the medicinal taste, making it easy to drink large amounts and potentially overdose.

The nickname "lean" reflects the need to lean against something for stability when high. The nicknames "red," "yellow," "green," or "purple" refer to the color of the cough syrup used, each offering a different high, with "red" considered the best.

Today, rap musicians continue to glamorize Lean, further increasing its abuse. This trend, combined with reduced prescribing after the opioid crisis was declared in 2017, has escalated the cost of codeine syrup on the black market. Pints of codeine-containing syrup can cost thousands of dollars. The exorbitant cost of "sippin' syrup" has made the habit a status symbol. But what happens to your character that can no longer afford Lean? Like so many others, he'll turn to the cheaper, easier-to-access oxycodone and a whole new list of dangerous risks (see "Oxycodone" in this chapter).

Sweet candy and soda mask the potency of Lean, making it easy to overdose.

Medically, codeine was a mainstay of cough and pain treatment for decades. However, in 2012, the Food and Drug Administration (FDA) reviewed numerous deaths in children treated with codeine after surgeries or for cough. Codeine must be metabolized to morphine in the body before it has any effect and genetics impact the rate of this process. Some people convert codeine too fast, causing rapid spikes in morphine blood levels, extreme sedation, and dangerously slow breathing. In children even up to 18 years old, this morphine spike can cause breathing to stop completely. By 2017, the FDA recommended not using codeine in children and some teens. This recommendation, together with restrictions due to the opioid crisis, caused a great reduction in codeine prescribing.

The high cost of codeine cough syrup can drive your character to abuse oxycodone instead.

If your story takes place before the warnings, your character could easily abuse the codeine prescribed for his child's cough or to control the pain after surgery, such as a tonsillectomy or an appendix removal. For plots taking place after the restrictions, getting that codeine will be more difficult for your character. He *could* find a bottle of codeine pills, left over from some previous prescription, buried in the back of the medicine cabinet. Now, *there's* a believable scene.

Slang Terms

(Since terminology and slang terms change over time, further research is highly encouraged.)

Street names

Captain Cody, Cody, doors and fours, little c, school boy, T3s or T4s (when combined with acetaminophen).

For Lean: dirty sprite, drank, green, red, yellow, purple, sizzurp, syrup, tussin

Other terms

- Kicking the cup: to stop the habit of drinking Lean, as in "He's been tryin' to kick the cup."
- Leaning on syrup: refers to a person drinking syrup, as in "I was leanin' pretty good last night."
- Sipping: drinking syrup, as in "He was sippin' red all night."

Weaving the Plot

How is it used?

Combination codeine/acetaminophen tablets and syrup have been prescribed for pain but are also abused for the opiate high. Codeine/promethazine syrups have been prescribed primarily for coughs. But abusers add that syrup to a mixture of soda and hard, flavored candy to make Lean. Your character might sip his Lean out of a set of double-stacked Styrofoam cups, which has become symbolic of the drink. He might pour Lean onto cigarettes or blunts to smoke, or even use it like a syrup over foods, such as pancakes. Depending on the historical timeline of your story, if codeine syrup is realistically available, your character could swig the sweet, pungent cough syrup right from the bottle.

Now you try it

> **Writing Prompt #1** Create a backstory for one of your characters who abuses codeine pills. How did the abuse start? Were they prescribed after surgery? Or stolen from a parent's medicine cabinet? (You'll use this background in Writing Prompt #2.)

How will my character act or feel?

Codeine will make your character drowsy and not able to think clearly. Stomach pain (often described as "being kicked in the stomach") is common, causing nausea and vomiting. Codeine causes a light-headed high, which goes away with regular use unless the dose is increased. This can cause a chronic codeine-abusing character to need progressively higher and higher doses to get the high he wants. Eventually, the dose needed to get high will also cause a dangerous drop in his breathing rate and, possibly, death.

Because the sweetness of Lean masks the potency, your character will keep sipping it throughout the evening, getting progressively intoxicated. At first, he'll be relaxed and happy. But with continued sipping, he'll be slurring his words, mentally foggy, yawning, sleepy, staggering, and leaning against the wall for stability. For an interesting twist, the promethazine in the cough syrup can cause hallucinations at high doses adding another dimension to the character's troubles (see chapter 6).

High doses of Lean can cause a character to hallucinate.

With high codeine doses, your character runs the risk of dangerously slow, shallow breathing. He'll become drowsy, confused, unsteady, and unable to focus on a conversation. If his breathing is slow enough, his fingertips and lips will turn blue gray and he'll pass out. His breathing can even slow to a stop. Without emergency help, he'll die. Even with medical care, if his breathing isn't restarted quickly enough, brain damage can lead to permanent disabilities (see the appendix).

Is the character also drinking alcohol? Alcohol magnifies the dangers of codeine, so the risk of your character not being able to breathe can happen at lower codeine doses. He may not make it to the next scene before he's found in his room, dead.

Withdrawal can occur after chronic codeine use, leaving your character with symptoms that feel similar to a bad case of the flu. He may have nausea, vomiting, diarrhea, severe muscle aches, runny eyes, and a drippy nose. He'll also be constantly yawning and suffer from insomnia. And if he doesn't control the vomiting and diarrhea, he can develop life-threatening dehydration, ending in heart failure and death. He'll be tempted to take codeine again to end his misery, but when he can't find any, he might move on to oxycodone or heroin (see "Oxycodone" or "Heroine" in this chapter).

Now you try it

> **Writing Prompt #2** Using the background from Writing Prompt #1, create a scene where your character is offered Lean at a party and decides to try it, not realizing how potent it is. How will the scene progress?

How long will this drug affect my character?

Pain or cough control from codeine can start in as little as fifteen to thirty minutes and last two to three hours. The euphoria, clumsiness, drowsiness, and mental fogginess from abuse starts in about fifteen minutes and slowly decreases over three to four hours. So, if your character is sipping Lean or popping codeine tablets all night, these symptoms will only start to fade after he takes that last dose.

PUTTING IT ALL TOGETHER

Sample Scenario The red lights are still flashing, as she frantically points the paramedics into her house and to her son on the bathroom floor. His body is motionless, his lips blue.

"He just fell. He wasn't breathing." Then she sees her bottle of pain pills on the floor, empty. "Oh, God! No!" she wails.

Now you try it

Writing Prompt #3 Have your character from Writing Prompt #2 grab the car keys and stagger toward the parking lot as the party is ending. How does the character act? How does this scene end? Will the character be stopped before driving off? Or will there be a deadly accident?

FENTANYL

Brief History/Social Context

Want to write a scene with a drug that will resonate with almost every reader in America? With the growing epidemic of fentanyl overdoses and the historic number of drug busts splashed across news headlines, fentanyl has become a household name.

Fentanyl is related to morphine, but instead of being extracted from the opium poppy plant, it's made in a lab (synthetic). Given that fentanyl is one hundred times more potent than morphine and fifty times more potent than heroin, today's headlines have rightfully made fentanyl a feared street drug. It's important to note that, when used correctly, *medical* fentanyl is a good and safe pain medicine that's been successfully used since it was developed in the 1950s.

So, if it can be used safely, what makes fentanyl so dangerous? It's because fentanyl is so potent that the difference between a safe and deadly dose is extremely small—in the magnitude of a few grains of salt! That means a small dose miscalculation can lead to a lethal mistake and medical errors do occur, despite

Storylines involving the risks of fentanyl will resonate with readers.

great caution. For example, calculation errors with fentanyl pain injections have led to death. Serious dosing errors with fentanyl pain patches have also been fatal, when the old patch wasn't removed before putting on a fresh one. Those used patches can still contain a lot of fentanyl, causing the patient to get dosed by both patches at the same time. Even discarded patches have led to unfortunate, deadly outcomes when toddlers have picked them out of the trash and used them as decorative body stickers.

These sad scenarios afford authors options for tragic character backstories—the grandpa who's grandchild died while visiting his house or the nurse who made a deadly error, losing her license and career. They also offer sinister plot twists—the antagonist who places several fentanyl patches on his victim.

Medical errors offer shockingly realistic plot twists.

But *most* fentanyl overdoses and deaths are caused by *illicit* (street) fentanyl. This is largely due to the huge quantities of fentanyl smuggled into the US and (unbeknownst to buyers) mixed by traffickers into other drugs, such as marijuana, heroin, and methamphetamine. Illicit fentanyl is also pressed into counterfeit oxycodone pills and stamped with brand-like symbols ("M" on one side, "30" on the other), making them look almost identical to real oxycodone tablets. In addition, fentanyl is being made into many other pills, such as counterfeit Xanax (alprazolam), Vicodin, and Adderall. In just 2022 *alone*, over fifty million fentanyl-containing pills and over 10,000 pounds of additional fentanyl powder were seized in the US, with a single pound of fentanyl powder able to make over 225,000 potentially lethal doses. It's estimated that the total amount of illicit fentanyl that's been confiscated is more than enough to kill every person in the US.

Why is fentanyl added to these other drugs if it can be so lethal? Fentanyl's a cheap additive that gives a bigger high, increasing sales and product demand. But the traffickers are not as concerned about mixing batches carefully, leaving some with little fentanyl, while others contain potentially lethal amounts. In fact, about 40 percent of counterfeit pills confiscated in the US in 2021 contained what are considered lethal amounts of fentanyl.

In contemporary fiction, a fentanyl overdose can befall your character using almost any street drug.

A small, but growing, number of these overdoses is due to a fentanyl cousin, carfentanil. This animal tranquilizer is one hundred times more potent than fentanyl. A dose the size of a single grain of salt can be lethal. Carfentanil became infamously tied to the 2002 Moscow theater hostage crisis involving Chechen terrorists. Tragically, after failed negotiations, the Russian military pumped an aerosolized combination of carfentanil, along with other potent chemicals, into the air vents of the crowded theater, resulting in the deaths of not only the terrorists but also 129 hostages. This same drug is being found in some batches of heroin, cocaine, and counterfeit pills.

Between 2022 and 2023, several other blends of fentanyl began appearing in the US, creating another wave of overdose deaths. Xylazine (Tranq) is a potent veterinary tranquilizer that's now considered the deadliest new additive to illicit drugs. It's not only been found in supplies of fentanyl but also heroin, methamphetamine, and cocaine. Xylazine is used to boost the high from these other drugs and to make the very short high from fentanyl last longer. But it can also cause a lethal drop in the user's blood pressure, heart rate, and breathing. And there is no antidote. Since xylazine isn't an opioid, naloxone cannot reverse these fatal effects (see chapter 3). In addition, xylazine causes skin abscesses that turn into rotting tissue that needs to be amputated to avoid death.

Xylazine-laced fentanyl may cause your character to die even after being given naloxone.

The current fentanyl situation in the US is considered a crisis. But fiction stories set in the 1990s can also involve the risks of fentanyl-tainted drugs. At that time, a street heroin called "Tango and Cash" contained fentanyl and led to many fatalities. About forty pounds of fentanyl was seized from the two clandestine labs making the Tango and Cash—enough to potentially kill over nine million people.

Fentanyl offers writers a variety of dangerous plot twists: a college student who buys "Adderall" to stay awake and cram for final exams may accidentally be taking a fentanyl-laced counterfeit; an addict dying of a fentanyl overdose after taking what he thought was his usual heroin hit (dose). But fentanyl also offers many nonlethal options to build character dimension: the homeless character seen in the subway inhaling fentanyl fumes wafting up from a crumpled piece of aluminum foil; your protagonist's elderly mother who uses fentanyl pain patches to keep her cancer pain at bay. And with a fentanyl vaccine currently being developed, the way fentanyl addiction can realistically be portrayed may soon change.

Fentanyl is a very concentrated and dangerous drug, but there are some scenes that authors should avoid writing. Don't include a character dying after touching fentanyl tablets or inhaling a small amount of fentanyl dust that's floating in the air. Erroneous information about these facts is readily available on the internet from typically well-respected resources. At the beginning of the fentanyl crisis, several of these resources circulated frightening information warning first responders and the general public that merely touching fentanyl tablets or inhaling airborne powder particles would bring rapid death. This misinformation escalated as other organizations, including media outlets, circulated these "facts," some adding them to training videos. However, in 2017, the American College of Medical Toxicology (ACMT) and the American Academy of Clinical Toxicology (AACT) published a position statement that debunked these myths. Yet, as of 2022, inaccurate information continues to be widely circulated. As an author, this means needing to critically assess all information from a variety of reputable resources in order to validate what is factual.

So . . . *can* your character plausibly die from inhaling fentanyl particles in the air? It's highly unlikely under most realistic scenarios. The ACMT/AACT report states that even in manufacturing plants that make fentanyl powder, it would take several hours of exposure without a safety mask to inhale the equivalent of a typical adult fentanyl dose. But, what about those tragic deaths in the Moscow theater hostage crisis? Those were not caused by fentanyl but the much more potent carfentanil, plus other powerful chemicals, and a unique aerosolized delivery method.

Creating an overdose scene with a character who just touches fentanyl is even less realistic. Fentanyl absorbs through the skin, but at an extremely slow rate. Even fentanyl pain patches take hours of continuous skin contact to begin to work.

Is it unrealistic for a character's flaw to be a fentanyl addiction? If it's so lethal, wouldn't my character just die? Not necessarily. Getting high on fentanyl can be done without taking a lethal dose. It's even realistic for your fentanyl (or even heroin) addict to seek out fentanyl-laced pills to fill his craving. How will your character know where to find a supply? Fentanyl users are often connected to suppliers already. But if not, he might just watch the local news. Reports of accidental fentanyl

Don't have your character die just from touching fentanyl tablets.

overdoses in the community will signal where nearby supplies can be found. He also might be able to order fentanyl through a social media app. Sellers working through these apps have devised an entire system of communication using special jargon and emojis, complete with menus, to convey how to get almost any street drug. Believe it or not, the app can even be used to have the order delivered, kind of like ordering a pizza. What an interesting scene that would make!

Fentanyl addiction from surgical anesthesia isn't realistic, but developing an addiction to pain pills is.

On the other hand, it would not be realistic to have a character become addicted to fentanyl after surgery. Addiction comes from the quick euphoric fentanyl rush that ends quickly, resulting in craving another high. But with surgery, the dose used is very controlled and doesn't cause that rush. However, it *would* be realistic to have your character become addicted to the pain pills he uses after that surgery. When his prescription runs out, it's believable for him seek out illicit pain pills. And what kind of pills is he likely to mistakenly buy? Those fentanyl-tainted counterfeit pain pills. See the great plot twist building?

Slang Terms

(Since terminology and slang terms change over time, further research is highly encouraged.)

Street names

- Fentanyl: Apache, bluies, blues, China girl, China white, dance fever, fetty, friend, goodfella, jackpot, TNT.
- Carfentanil: drop dead, elephant tranqs, 80's.
- Xylazine and fentanyl blend: tranq, tranq dope, sleep-cut, Philly, dope, zombie drug (also used for bath salts).

Other terms

- Gray death: a mixture of heroin plus fentanyl (or a fentanyl cousin, like carfentanil); also increasingly refers to an inconsistent mixture containing a variety of opioids.
- Tango and Cash: a brand of heroin increasingly tainted with forms of fentanyl.

How is it used?

Medically, fentanyl is often given as a slow injection or intravenous infusion. It's important not to have a character rapidly inject the fentanyl into a patient (like a quick push into a vein)—unless he's the villain. This scene may seem appropriately dramatic, but in reality, rapid injection can quickly make the person's chest muscles become rigid, making breathing difficult or impossible and causing asphyxia if not quickly reversed. Fentanyl's also sometimes given as a nose spray for sedation. For chronic pain, such as cancer, skin patches may be used and must be replaced about every three days. Fentanyl also comes as a sublingual (under the tongue) spray and a berry-flavored lollipop for breakthrough pain. It'll be important to research which of these forms of fentanyl is available during your story's historical timeline since the products change rapidly.

Abuse and addiction scenarios with fentanyl include many options. A character can inject it to get high. He can scrape the fentanyl gel out of the skin patches to smoke, swallow, or inject. Or, he might either chew on a patch or brew it like tea to get high. Keep in mind, your character won't really know how much drug he's taking when manipulating a patch, even if he's done it before. *This time he might get high, he might overdose, or he might die.*

> **Chewing fentanyl patches could get your character high or kill him.**

Illicit blue fentanyl pills are easy to get and popular to abuse. They can be swallowed or crushed to snort or smoke. Experienced abusers know they can't be certain of the amount of fentanyl in each pill. Because of the risk, they may decide to swallow, snort, or inject only part of a tablet, hoping the portion used isn't deadly. Out of desperation, some addicts use the entire tablet, willing to take the risk for the effect.

Medical use of carfentanil is primarily by veterinarians as a tranquilizer for large animals (like elephants). When abused, it's too potent to use alone, so it's generally blended into other drugs or added to counterfeit pills.

Now you try it

> **Writing Prompt #1** Choose one of your characters to ask a friend for some pain pills. Who's the character and why are the pills needed? (You'll use this background in Writing Prompt #2.)

How will my character act or feel?

In medical doses, fentanyl will cause relaxation, drowsiness, decreased pain, and possibly a mild euphoria (except for the patches). If your character is abusing fentanyl, you can depict him as very relaxed, light-headed, mentally foggy, and drowsy. He'll speak slowly and stagger if he walks. He may nod off to sleep in the middle of talking to someone. Want a disturbing side effect? Opioids, like fentanyl, can make some people hallucinate spiders or bugs crawling on their skin or on nearby objects, like the wall, even at normal doses.

Rapidly injected fentanyl doses can make your character's chest muscles rigid within a minute or two, making it difficult or impossible to breathe. Dubbed "wooden chest syndrome," your character's muscles should look tense and his lips should start turning blue. For added drama, he could realistically have a seizure, with his muscles convulsing and foam dripping from his clenched jaws. But even if the character injects the fentanyl carefully, a high dose can still cause dangerously slow (or stopped) breathing within a few minutes. This risk is even higher if he's been drinking alcohol or taking sedatives, like a benzodiazepine (see chapter 14). Either way, without air your character will soon pass out, his lips turning bluish, and death may soon occur unless the antidote, naloxone, is given in time (see chapter 3). Even with an emergency dose of naloxone, if his breathing isn't restored soon enough, he may suffer permanent disabilities from brain damage (see the appendix).

Rapidly injecting fentanyl is dramatic, but can make breathing impossible.

If your plot involves a villain secretly hiding several fentanyl patches on your protagonist, don't have the character develop symptoms right away. It'll take hours before enough fentanyl absorbs across the skin before the character begins to become progressively drowsier. Is this when your character begins to realize something is wrong? As he desperately feels around his body, looking for the cause, your readers will be stressing, wondering what will happen. If he doesn't find the patches in time, his breathing can slow enough that he becomes delirious. Perhaps your character's fingers find the patches and he rips them off just as his vision begins to blur. Then, as he struggles to see the figure entering the room, everything goes black. Without an urgent dose of the antidote, naloxone, this character will probably not survive the scene (see "Naloxone" in chapter 3). Why?

Because the fentanyl already in his skin will keep absorbing even after the patches are removed. Naloxone doses can help him breathe again. But don't have him get just one dose of antidote, then wake up, and escape. As long as that fentanyl is still absorbing, he'll need a few more doses of the antidote over the next several hours to be safe.

The effects from fentanyl skin patches don't stop the instant they are removed.

Carfentanil is so potent that if it's mixed into a character's drugs, he can realistically suffer a rapidly lethal overdose. He'll be dizzy, with clammy skin, and find breathing difficult. As his breathing shuts down, he'll pass out and possibly have a seizure. Without oxygen, he'll die in a matter of minutes. If he injects a drug that's been laced with carfentanil, you can convincingly declare him unconscious within a few seconds and dead soon thereafter, as his breathing will come to an abrupt stop.

Tranq dope will put a character into imminent peril, whether injected, swallowed, or snorted. He'll rapidly be staggering, his vision blurry. As his breathing slows, he can fall to the ground with a seizure, his body convulsing and foam dripping from his mouth. His breathing can then slow to a halt. But when your character gets a rescue dose of naloxone, the opioid antidote, it won't work. Naloxone will only reverse the breathing effects of whatever opioid was mixed into the xylazine. But the xylazine *itself* arrests breathing—and naloxone doesn't work on this drug. Your character is going to need an emergency medical team to put a breathing tube down his throat and get him to a hospital, or he's going to die.

Withdrawal will create misery for your fentanyl-addicted character within a few hours of his last dose. He'll feel like he has a very bad case of the flu, with severe muscle aches and pains, runny eyes and nose, profuse sweating, poor sleep, nausea, vomiting, and diarrhea. He'll also be agitated and anxious, with drug cravings. Withdrawal symptoms can worsen over a few days before symptoms gradually start to improve. He can survive withdrawal, unless his vomiting and diarrhea are severe enough to cause life-threatening dehydration that leads to heart failure and death.

Withdrawal from fentanyl may not be lethal, but the severe dehydration from vomiting and diarrhea can be.

Does your character inject fentanyl? He can develop infected injection sites (such as along his forearm) or a life-threatening heart infection. Contracting HIV (Human

Immunodeficiency Virus) or hepatitis from sharing used needles with other drug abusers is also a realistic risk. If the fentanyl is mixed with xylazine, he'll likely develop painful sores at his injection sites that quickly decay to the point of needing an amputation to avoid death.

Now you try it

> **Writing Prompt #2** Continue the scene from Writing Prompt #1. The character has taken one of the pills, which turns out to contain fentanyl. You get to decide if it's a lethal dose or not. How does the character feel? How does this scene unfold? End the scene with a page-turner.

How long will this drug affect my character?

Pain control from injected fentanyl starts within two to three minutes and lasts for up to two hours. The rush of euphoria from abused fentanyl starts within seconds when injected, smoked, or snorted. The high can last as long as two hours or as short as thirty minutes. In an overdose scene, don't have your character instantly drop dead. Instead, life-threatening effects should evolve over several minutes. For example, his breathing can become very slow and eventually come to a halt. Death can be more rapid in a character that's also been drinking alcohol or taking sedatives (see chapter 14). With swallowed tablets, fentanyl must first be absorbed in the stomach, so your character might not feel effects for several minutes. For fentanyl patches, it takes about three to four hours for enough drug to absorb across the skin for effects to begin. This is true no matter how many patches are used. Your evil villain that puts several patches on his victim will be long gone when the first signs of danger appear. When the patches are removed, the drug reservoir that's still in the skin will continue to cause effects for several more hours. The victim's rescuer will need to give him the antidote, naloxone, several times over the next few hours to prevent death (see "A Word about Antidotes" in chapter 3).

Carfentanil has only been tested in animals, so facts about how long it lasts in people are lacking. But, in general, the time from injection to being unconscious can be as short as a few seconds, with death soon after from a lack of oxygen. An emergency dose of the antidote, naloxone, is needed for your character to survive (see "A Word about Antidotes" in chapter 3). Because the antidote wears off faster than the carfentanil, deadly symptoms can return and your character will need more doses of naloxone over the next few hours until all the danger has passed.

Sample Scenario #1 Kasey reaches into the garbage, smirking. Grandpa's always good for a fentanyl patch. He pops it into his mouth, chewing it on the way back to his room. He props himself on his pillows, enjoying the gentle buzz in his head. When he looks up, the room is slowly spinning. *It didn't hit this hard last time.* The room feels hot, his chest tight. *Something's wrong.* He grabs at his chest, spits out the patch, and gasps for air. "Grandpa?" he calls, but his voice is weak, faint. His eyelids close, his body goes limp.

Sample Scenario #2 She holds still, watching Terry tap her vein, wincing slightly at the pinch of the needle, then sighs at the familiar rush.

"Good?" he asks.

"Shit, yeah." She smiles, letting her body relax, watching as he sticks his own arm, then sits next to her. After a few minutes, bitter vomit rushes to her throat and she leans over, letting it splash to the floor. She grabs for Terry, but his body falls sideways. He's not moving. Her head spins, then the room goes dark.

Sample Scenario #3 He crushes the little blue pill into the scrap of foil he dug from the trash. His fingers fumble with the lighter, then he holds the flame against the powder. He leans into the smoke, cupping a shaking hand to drive the fumes toward his nose, and takes a deep breath.

Now you try it

Writing Prompt #3 Pick one of your characters to have an addiction to fentanyl. Write a scene where the character is suffering from withdrawal. How does the character feel? Act? Interact with others? How does this scene end?

HEROIN

Brief History/Social Context

Heroin (diacetylmorphine) is well known as a highly addictive opioid and is made from the morphine that's extracted from opium poppy plants. First developed in the late 1800s, it was, like many abused drugs, initially used as

Heroin could have been used to treat your character's cough in the early 1900s.

a medical treatment. You may be surprised to know it was even temporarily marketed under the name "Heroin" as a treatment for cough and respiratory illness.

But with the potent euphoria and severe drug cravings caused by heroin, addiction and overdoses quickly escalated. Because addiction was so widespread by 1924, it became illegal to import, manufacture, or possess heroin in the US. That didn't stop abuse, however, and heroin continued to be smuggled into the country. Interestingly, in the 1960s, a government crackdown on heroin pivoted many users temporarily to opium abuse (see "Opium" in this chapter). However, heroin use has continued fairly undeterred. In 2021, almost one million Americans reported using heroin in the previous year. Since then, the number of heroin users has grown, in part as an unintended consequence of the reduced prescribing of pain pills due to the opioid crisis. Decreased prescribing has led to less opioids, like oxycodone, being funneled into street drug supplies, resulting in some users initially turning to heroin and more recently to counterfeit oxycodone and fentanyl. But don't have your character that takes a few pain pills (like oxycodone or Vicodin) after his surgery suddenly become an addict that turns to heroin use. The same is true if he gets fentanyl or morphine for pain during that surgery. But while most people treated for a short time with an opioid do not become heroin addicts, the majority of heroin users started their journey to addiction through the use of other opioids, such oxycodone. Heroin abuse isn't just for adult characters, either. Your protagonist may have friends in his high school that started using heroin when pain pills became harder to buy.

Previous abuse of opioid pain pills, such as Vicodin or oxycodone, is a realistic backstory for your character's journey to heroin addiction.

What makes heroin such a popular drug to abuse? It can be snorted or smoked, avoiding the stigma associated with injecting drugs. Unfortunately, this can make heroin seem safer, tempting your character that might otherwise not try an illicit drug. However, whether snorted, smoked, or injected, the potent high from heroin makes it incredibly addictive. Heroin is also fairly cheap and easy to buy due to the large supply in the US.

There are many dangers awaiting a character using heroin. Even with his first use, he risks overdosing on this potent opioid, causing him to suffer dangerously slow (or stopped) breathing, seizures, a coma, and possibly death. Your character could also suffer a stroke or heart attack if his heroin has been cut (diluted) with the cheap additives traffickers use to extend their supplies and profits, such as sugar, starch, or powdered milk. These additives can clump in your character's veins when he injects his hit (dose), blocking blood flow and leading to a stroke or heart attack. Even more dangerous is the trend of heroin tainted with fentanyl to boost the intensity of the high and increase demand. If the heroin contains fentanyl, this scene can suddenly pivot from his expected high to a lethal fentanyl overdose (see "Fentanyl" in this chapter).

Slang Terms

(Since terminology and slang terms change over time, further research is highly encouraged.)

Street names

black (black tar), brown sugar (brownish heroin), China white (white heroin), H, hell dust, Henry, hero, horse, junk, ska, smack, thunder, train

Other terms

- Chasing the Dragon: smoking heroin or inhaling heroin vapor.
- Gray death: a mixture of heroin plus either fentanyl or a fentanyl cousin, like carfentanil. Increasingly, it may be an inconsistent mix of a variety of opioids.
- Speedballing: mixing an opioid together with a stimulant, such as combining heroin with cocaine. These can be mixed into the same syringe or may be injected one right after the other.

Weaving the Plot

How is it used?

Depending on the process used, heroin can be a white, brown, or black powder. Or, it can be a sticky black substance called "black tar heroin." In general, heroin can be injected, snorted, or smoked, but may need to be manipulated first. For example, injecting heroin requires that the powder first be dissolved, heated, and filtered (often through a cotton ball or something similar). It can be shot into a vein (mainlined, slammed), into a muscle (muscled), or injected just under the skin (popped). Powdered heroin can be simply snorted or diluted in a small amount of water before spraying up the nose. But black tar heroin is such a sticky substance that it's difficult to simply crush and snort. Users have various ways to harden the tar to make crushing easier, such as freezing it temporarily. Smoking heroin can simply be done after sprinkling the powder onto a cigarette (either tobacco or marijuana). It can also be placed on a piece of foil and heated, with the fumes directed toward the nose using a straw or cupped hands.

Now you try it

> **Writing Prompt #1** Write a scene in which one of your characters walks in on a friend that's in the middle of taking a heroin hit (dose). What does the character see? How does your character react? (You'll continue this scene in Writing Prompt #2.)

How will my character act or feel?

Heroin causes a rapid euphoric rush (high) and a wave of pleasurable feelings. The high has been described as feeling like being cradled in a warm blanket. Your character will be filled with tranquility and feel as if all his problems have been washed away. If he injects heroin, this rush will start within seconds, followed by drowsiness and the sense his body has become very heavy. If smoking or snorting heroin, the rush won't be quite as intense since the effects start more slowly. Either way, his mind will be foggy, his mouth dry, and his itchy skin will be warm and flushed. As the quick rush fades, your character can experience a phenomenon called "being on the nod," going in and out of consciousness, nodding off to sleep and then reawakening. This can continue for an hour or two before he rests for several hours in a trance-like state.

Your character can "be on the nod" for an hour or two after his heroin hit.

Is this one of your character's first few times using heroin? He won't enjoy it as much as he hoped. Along with that incredibly pleasant rush, a newcomer can have severe stomach discomfort and nausea. He may vomit just once or repeatedly for hours, ending in dry heaves. It can take several heroin experiences before his body begins to adapt and vomiting becomes less problematic. But the rush from that first heroin high will have been so wonderful that he'll keep using heroin hoping to get that same intense rush again. But it will become the big lie he chases. Subsequent heroin highs are rarely as strong as the first one and can become less intense with each use. Trying to get that elusive high will feed your character's addiction and offer you plenty of conflicts for the plot.

There are many other risks with heroin. Does your character inject it? He can develop infections ranging from sores at injection sites (like along his forearm) to a life-threatening heart infection. Or the character can contract a blood-carried disease, such as hepatitis or HIV, from sharing needles with other drug abusers. Does he snort heroin? He can develop a hole in the tissue between his nostrils. And after chronic heroin use, permanent changes to his brain chemicals can cause depression and antisocial behavior. If your protagonist is a female, she may stop having regular menstrual cycles.

Your character can be driven by the unattainable desire of experiencing the intensity of that first heroin high again.

How fast will your character become addicted to heroin? Pretty fast! After just a few doses, he'll develop a deep desire to relive that rush. Even without that intense high, each hit of heroin will trigger the pleasure centers of his brain so strongly that addiction will quickly develop. Intense hunger for more heroin will create a desperate cycle. The cravings and fear of painful withdrawal symptoms will drive extreme drug-seeking behavior. *Now* your character will do *anything*, no matter the consequences, to get another hit.

Heroin addiction can happen rapidly after just a few doses.

Your protagonist can wake up in the morning feeling "dope sick" and needing more heroin to stave off the beginnings of withdrawal. which start just six to twelve hours after a dose. He'll feel horrible, with body aches and pains. If he doesn't get another fix (dose) soon he'll be shivering, his skin covered in goosebumps, and his clothes will be drenched from a cold sweat. His eyes and nose will be running and he'll be suffering from stomach cramps, nausea, vomiting, and diarrhea. Painful muscle spasms will cause uncontrollable leg movements. In fact, these symptoms were the origins of the terms *cold turkey* (goose bumps) and *kicking the habit* (leg movements). At this point, your character will be desperate for another hit. He may even steal to get the money for more heroin and then beg for used syringes from another addict. If he doesn't find more heroin, he'll survive the ordeal, although his withdrawal will continue to get worse over several days and may last a week. But if his diarrhea and vomiting are bad enough, your character risks dying from life-threatening effects caused by severe dehydration.

Your character can wake up dope sick, desperate to get another hit of heroin and end the misery of withdrawal.

If your character has been using heroin regularly, he can become tolerant, meaning he'll need higher doses to get his high. At some point the dose he needs will contain enough heroin to cause an overdose. He might also overdose if he gets more potent heroin than he expects or takes his usual dose after he has gone through a drug rehabilitation program. Your character can suffer dangerously slow (or stopped) breathing, blueish lips and fingernails, and a very slow heartbeat. He'll pass out. If he suffers a seizure, he may have foam dripping from his clenched jaws as his body convulses. Death will follow without emergency medical help. Naloxone, an antidote for opioid overdose, can save your character from dying if it's given in time (see "A Word about Antidotes in chapter 3). Even with the naloxone, if his breathing isn't restarted quickly enough, your character can be left with permanent disabilities from brain damage (see the appendix).

> **Your character can overdose from heroin that's more potent than usual.**

Now you try it

> **Writing Prompt #2** Continue the scene from Writing Prompt #1. Let the friend reveal how the heroin addiction began, after the grogginess from the hit wears off. How does your character respond? Does this revelation affect their relationship?

How long will this drug affect my character?

The intense rush from injected heroin starts almost immediately, while smoking it causes a delayed, less intense rush in about twenty to thirty seconds. The high from snorting heroin starts subtly over about five to ten minutes. For an hour or two, your character may float in and out of consciousness ("be on the nod") followed by another hour or two in a trance-like state, with mild drowsiness and a sense of well-being.

PUTTING IT ALL TOGETHER

> **Sample Scenario** He walked into the bedroom and stopped. "You said you weren't using anymore," he snapped, walking to the bed. He glared at her, slumped on the bed, an empty syringe next to her, a bag of powder on the table.
> She mumbled something and reached toward him.
> He slapped her hand away. "The baby's right in the next room. What the *hell* were you thinking?"

Now you try it

Writing Prompt #3 Write a scene from the point of view of the heroin user in Writing Prompt #2. It's several days later. The character ran out of heroin and money yesterday. How does the character feel? What happens next?

HYDROMORPHONE (DILAUDID)

Brief History/Social Context

Hydromorphone (Dilaudid) is about eight times stronger than morphine and was originally marketed in the mid-1930s to treat pain (see "A Note of Caution: Using Brand Names" in chapter 1). Unfortunately, because it causes a potent euphoria, abuse escalated from the 1960s and only recently declined due to the availability of cheap oxycodone. Abusers inject (bang), eat (swallow), and snort hydromorphone for an intense high described as a deep sense of extreme relaxation while being wrapped in a warm blanket.

Some people seek out more hydromorphone after initially experiencing the euphoria from a dose in an emergency room or after surgery, resulting in abuse and eventual addiction. In fact, it's realistic to have your character go to an emergency room (ER) complaining of severe pain in an attempt to get another dose. This happens enough in some ERs that they no longer prescribe hydromorphone. It's also realistic to have your character "doctor shop," visiting different doctors until he finds one that will prescribe hydromorphone. However, this has become much more challenging since the opioid crisis was declared in 2017, resulting in restriction of opioid prescribing. In addition, suspicious doctors can check an online database listing all the controlled drugs that a patient has been prescribed, making doctor shopping difficult. When that ER doctor won't give him any hydromorphone, your character can simply use a social media app to find someone who will.

> Your character might fake severe pain in an ER in an attempt to get a dose of hydromorphone.

Hydromorphone is often abused as an injection (IV) after crushing the pellets from the extended-release capsules and diluting them in liquid (a wash). Some users will inject all the diluted drug for an extreme high, but they risk an overdose, since each capsule contains a full day's dose of hydromorphone. So, to avoid this risk

Diluted hydromorphone might be shared by your character with other users to keep the costs down.

(and because the capsules are very expensive), the prepared liquid may be shared among several addicts. In this case, your character may share the syringe with other users, each taking a turn dipping the needle into the wash, injecting their hit, and passing the syringe to the next user. This way, everyone shares in the cost. Unfortunately, they also share in the risk of developing infections, such as hepatitis or HIV.

Like any opioid, hydromorphone in high doses can be lethal. Your character's breathing will become dangerously slow (or completely stop). He can have a seizure, pass out, and die from a lack of oxygen without emergency help.

Your character can also suffer withdrawal.

Street Terms

(Since terminology and slang terms change over time, further research is highly encouraged.)

Street names

D, dillies, dust, footballs, juice, and smack

Weaving the Plot

How is it used?

Medical hydromorphone comes as tablets, capsules, liquids, and an injection. If regular tablets are being abused, they may be eaten (swallowed), crushed and snorted, plugged (inserted into the rectum) or, more often, dissolved to inject (slam, bang). *Extended-release* tablets are snorted or diluted before injecting for an intense high, but, since this releases an entire day's dose of drug all at once, it also risks a fatal overdose. To avoid the risk, your character may instead keep the dilution for several doses or, because of the high cost of hydromorphone, share it among several people. The diluted solution can be dipped into with a syringe, injected, and then the syringe passed to the next person. When injecting, your character will wait to see a tiny bit of blood (flash) in his syringe to assure he's in a vein, before pushing the plunger.

Now you try it

> **Writing Prompt #1** Develop a scene for a character that's house sitting for an out-of-town friend. The character finds hydromorphone tablets in the medicine cabinet and decides to experiment with snorting them. What makes the character decide to do this? Stop the scene just as the last line is snorted. (You'll continue this scene in Writing Prompt #2.)

How will my character act or feel?

Hydromorphone causes a rapid, floating sense of deep relaxation. Your character will be flooded with warm, pleasurable feelings, alternating with bouts of drowsiness. His mouth will be dry, and he'll have trouble thinking clearly. He might be nauseous and possibly vomit.

Are you writing an overdose scene? Your character's mind will be foggy, he'll be confused, dizzy, and feel weak. He'll be clumsy and stagger if he walks. His skin will become cold and clammy. He might pass out or fall to the floor from a seizure, with foam coming from his mouth as his body convulses. His breathing will become very slow or stop, causing a bluish tinge to his lips and fingernails. If his breathing isn't restarted quickly enough, brain damage can leave him with permanent disabilities (see the appendix).

Withdrawal can cause your character to feel like he's suffering from the flu. He may be drenched with sweat and suffering painful muscle aches, tremors (shakes), nausea, vomiting, severe diarrhea, runny eyes, and a dripping nose. He'll also yawn quite often and struggle with insomnia. He'll survive withdrawal, unless he develops life-threatening dehydration from the vomiting and diarrhea.

Now you try it

> **Writing Prompt #2** Continue the scene from Writing Prompt #1. How will the character act after snorting hydromorphone? Want to add a twist? Is the character just starting to enjoy the high, when there's a jingle of keys at the front door as the owner arrives home early from the trip? And is the white residue from snorting still clinging to the character's nose?

How long will this drug affect my character?

Pain can be reduced for three to four hours after taking regular hydromorphone pills or the injection. Extended-release capsules can keep pain at bay for twelve to twenty-four hours. The high from swallowing regular pills will start in ten to twenty minutes and continue in waves, alternating with bouts of sleepiness. The extended-release tablets, however, have a slower start to the high when they're swallowed whole, lasting up to twenty-four hours, as the beads inside the capsule slowly release their contents. With snorting, the high can take five to ten minutes to begin. Injecting can cause a rapid high in less than a minute. The lightheaded, floating euphoria can disappear after thirty minutes.

PUTTING IT ALL TOGETHER

Sample Scenario Terry crushed the capsule inside the paper coffee cup and tossed in some water. His hands shook as he held the lighter under the cup, hoping it wouldn't catch on fire. He put the cup down and filled his syringe with the liquid, then looked for a fresh spot to jab the needle. He finally sank the needle into his arm, watching for the flash of red blood. Nothing. He pulled the needle out and tried again. This time he felt it slip into a vein, saw the little red flash, and shoved the plunger down. He hadn't even pulled the needle out before his head started swimming and he felt all his stress floating away.

Now you try it

Writing Prompt #3 Write a scene for one of your characters who's been taking hydromorphone for chronic pain since a car accident over a year ago. Now, the doctor won't prescribe anymore. Not only is withdrawal starting but the pain is coming back. How will your character react to the situation?

DESOMORPHINE (KROKODIL)

Brief History/Social Context

Looking for an incredibly deadly and addictive drug that can rot your character's skin? Krokodil is a great option. Dubbed the "drug that eats junkies," krokodil causes the user's skin to resemble grayish-green crocodile skin with bleeding wounds that eventually decay, exposing bone. This drug is not a good choice if you expect your character to survive, however, as life expectancy is a mere two years after the first dose.

Don't expect your character to live long if he starts using krokodil.

Krokodil was originally researched in the mid-1900s as a potential alternative to its cousin, morphine. When the magnitude of krokodil addiction was realized (it's worse than heroin), research was quickly abandoned. In 2004, a homemade version of krokodil gained popularity in Russia among heroin addicts. Unlike the original drug, this dangerous homebrew was a mixture of cheap codeine, hydrochloric acid, gasoline, red phosphate from matchbooks, and other toxic ingredients. It takes about thirty minutes to cook a batch of krokodil. With the short-lived high and intense drug cravings, users rotate cooking duties, creating a vicious cycle: cook, inject, get high, and repeat. It would be realistic to have several krokodil addicts sharing a rundown apartment, some passed out, some cooking, some agonizingly waiting for their next high, all on a path to a painful death.

Intense cravings will drive your character's behavior, despite bleeding wounds and rotting flesh.

By 2009, krokodil gained international attention because of its devastating effects. It was abused primarily in Russia and Ukraine, but Canada, Germany, and a handful of other European countries also reported cases. In 2013, a few cases of tissue decay in US drug abusers were initially thought to be from injected krokodil. The cases turned out to be from severely infected drug-injection sites and not from krokodil. Although periodic cases have continued to be reported, krokodil has never become popular in the US, since access to codeine is strictly regulated and heroin has remained inexpensive and readily available.

If your story is set in the US, don't be too fast to discount the idea of using krokodil as part of your plot. Today, heroin is cheap and codeine is difficult to access due to legal restrictions. But that can change. A good example is how it only took a few years for fentanyl to replace opioid pain pills, like oxycodone, as one of the leading causes of drug overdoses in the US. This was, in part, an unintended consequence of opioid prescribing restrictions enacted in response to the opioid crisis. It's easy to see a scenario where a government crackdown has not only created a heroin shortage but reduced the availability of cheap alternatives, such as fentanyl. With some creativity, something similar to krokodil could be the alternative. Surprisingly, krokodil is not the only flesh-eating drug option for plotting. In 2023, xylazine (a veterinary tranquilizer) was found in supplies of various of street drugs, such as fentanyl. Nicknamed Tranq dope, this deadly blend was leaving users with rotting wounds and creating a new wave of overdose deaths (see "Fentanyl" in this chapter).

Slang Terms

(Since terminology and slang terms change over time, further research is highly encouraged.)

Street names

crocodile, krokodil, Russian magic

Weaving the Plot

How is it used?

Krokodil is injected and the doses are repeated regularly to regain the intense high and avoid withdrawal.

Now you try it

> **Writing Prompt #1** A character with a heroin addiction is finding it harder to get a drug fix. Develop a scene where the character is offered krokodil, a new drug with a "better high." (You'll continue this scene in Writing Prompt #2.)

How will my character act or feel?

Krokodil causes a rapid, intense high and powerful pain numbing. Your character will realistically pass out while high. When he wakes, it's possible he'll already have cravings for more drug, even after his first dose. After only a few uses, without more he'll suffer withdrawal symptoms, like vomiting, body aches, painful muscles spasms, sweats, and unbearable cravings. With the all-consuming act of cooking krokodil and getting high, he won't be able to work, eventually running out of money for more drugs and food. To support his habit, he may have to turn to robbery. Skin wounds will develop at the krokodil injection

Krokodil will leave your character with rotting flesh that must be amputated to avoid death.

sites. As the injection sites worsen they'll become infected, painful, and turn grayish-green. He may not feel the wounds while he's high, since krokodil has such potent pain reducing effects. Eventually, the discolored skin will peel off, leaving bloody wounds and rotting tissue, exposing his bones. Without urgent treatment, these wounds can develop gangrene and the limb must be amputated before severe infection and death occurs. With a life expectancy of only two years, your character isn't likely to live long enough to develop infections such as hepatitis and HIV from sharing needles with other drug abusers.

Now you try it

> **Writing Prompt #2** Continue the scene from Writing Prompt #1, beginning just after your character wakes from the first krokodil high. What kind of thoughts, feelings, and fears does the character have? What happens next?

How long will this drug affect my character?

The intense high can start in as few as two to three minutes, wearing off within two hours.

PUTTING IT ALL TOGETHER

> **Sample Scenario** Trash and empty syringes litter the room. Bodies lay unconscious, strewn about the furniture, the floor. A woman sits slumped over a desk moaning, her swollen shoulder oozing reddish-green pus. Not far from her, a man hunches over a pot, stirring, his hand shaking. Bleeding sores cover his arms.
> "How much longer," moans the woman. "I need it *now*."

Now you try it

> **Writing Prompt #3** Continue with your character from Writing Prompt #2. Develop a scene that begins two weeks later. Your character is now addicted to krokodil and desperate for money to buy more. What happens when the character runs into an old friend outside of a grocery store?

METHADONE

Brief History/Social Context

Methadone is an opioid related to morphine and fentanyl that has been used since the 1940s. It's best known as an opioid withdrawal treatment, although it's also used for some kinds of pain. Methadone masks the unpleasant withdrawal symptoms of opioid addiction for twenty-four hours or more without causing a high when properly dosed.

Unfortunately, methadone is also abused. Because of this, prescribing and dispensing methadone is strictly regulated. Local pharmacies are currently only able to dispense methadone when it's specifically used for pain. Withdrawal doses must be dispensed from a specially certified outpatient treatment program (OTP) clinic and must usually be taken under observation because of the risk of doses being taken home to sell.

Clinics are required to screen clients for stringent requirements of admission, such as documented addiction for over a year, being incarcerated, or being pregnant. There are also requirements to prove the patient's stable, such as having a job and a place to live. Unfortunately, some patients being treated with methadone report suffering a social stigma by being on an opioid, with some housing units refusing them as tenants, making it difficult to continue to meet the requirements. The requirements also make it difficult or impossible for most homeless addicts, often without jobs, to qualify for treatment from OTPs.

Your character will have to meet OTP requirements to be realistically depicted as being treated with methadone for opioid addiction.

Your character will also face many challenges, assuming the program accepts her. She'll have to go to the OTP *every day* to get her next dose, often for months, before being allowed to go less frequently. She may have to drive a long way to get to the nearest clinic each day or take a bus across town, if the bus is even running. She'll face limited clinic hours and wait in a long line for hours with other clients waiting for doses. Depending on where the OTP is located, the others in line may be high or drunk and prone to starting physical fights if they are denied their dose because of a rule infraction (such as being drunk or high at the clinic).

A large part of your character's day may be spent getting to the OTP and back.

The character may be subjected to giving a urine sample in front of a worker for a drug test before being approved for her dose. When your exhausted character finally takes her dose, an employee will have to watch her swallow it to ensure she won't just take it home to sell. While she's at the clinic she may be treated with respect by the staff or feel like she's being judged. She's already had a full day, but your character now needs to get to work on time or take care of her children—whatever her daily obligations entail. And the next day, she'll repeat the process. To make life more challenging, by the time she arrives at her clinic appointment the next day, her dose may have already started wearing off, leaving her feeling shaky and nauseous.

How long will this go on for your stressed character trying to win the battle against her opioid addiction? Opioid treatment programs can last *months to years*, so your character will be dealing with this lifestyle for a long time—possibly for the rest of her life, since methadone can be very difficult, if not impossible, to stop taking. There's some hope for her overburdened schedule, however. As her treatment progresses, she'll slowly gain the privilege of "take-home" doses—at first one dose a week, then months later, two doses a week. These doses allow her to skip an appointment for those days she has a dose at home. It's a slow process to gain freedom, however. Eventually, she might be allowed to take home several doses a week. To get and keep this privilege, she'll have to pass random drug screens along the way and, in some cases, unannounced dose counts of her supply of take-home doses to make sure she hasn't been selling them.

Don't have your character suddenly be "clean" from heroin a month after starting a methadone program.

Since 2020, because of COVID-19, treatment clinics have allowed more take-home doses, even up to a three weeks' supply, depending on how stable and trustworthy the client is deemed. Telemedicine visits have also replaced some mandatory in-person clinic visits.

Because of all the barriers to the OTP treatment, it's very believable to have your character quit the program. It'll be easier to take her heroin or oxycodone. Or, she may stay in the program to be able to sell a few of her take-home doses to buy heroin instead.

Isn't there *something* easier than this for my character's withdrawal treatment? Well, yes and no. Several other drugs are used for opioid withdrawal, but they all come with inconveniences, prolonged treatment, or the risk of abuse. If your character can't get to daily OTP treatment, she might qualify for withdrawal treatment by a local physician that has undergone special training. This gives her much broader access to treatment and much less impact on her daily life. She won't be treated with methadone, though. Instead, she may be treated with either buprenorphine (Subutex) or a combination drug of buprenorphine with naloxone (Suboxone). Buprenorphine is a type of opioid and naloxone is an abuse deterrent added to help block a high. Legal changes in 2023 made this drug option available to a wider number of physicians wanting to treat withdrawal at their regular patient clinics, helping to get rid of one more barrier to care. Treatment doses can be sent home and your character will only need to go to the doctor's office every couple of days to be monitored.

But there's a catch. To start treatment on either of these drugs, your character needs to stop whatever opioid she's been abusing long enough to have withdrawal begin. Otherwise, these treatment drugs themselves can cause a rapid and severe withdrawal, as they compete with the effects of any other opioid in the body. Your character will be miserable before starting treatment or she may fall victim to her cravings for a high.

Unfortunately, these treatment drugs are also abused. Users may inject or snort them. And despite the abuse deterrent in Suboxone, some users claim they're able to get a high, despite the euphoria not being as intense as desired. Abuse is bad enough that there's an entire culture of "Sub" abuse. Partial doses are taken to stave off withdrawal until the user can get a fix of heroin. Or doses may be stocked away and sold or exchanged for other illicit drugs. Users also describe the withdrawal from these drugs as worse than what they experienced from heroin.

Delineating all the nuances to opioid withdrawal treatment and the various drug programs is far beyond the scope of this book—the subject could make an entire book by itself! Authors can find out more regarding these various programs and the drugs by using the search terms *certification of OTPs*, *buprenorphine opioid withdrawal*, or *methadone opioid withdrawal*.

Pain treatment with methadone didn't begin until the mid-1970s; before then, it could only be prescribed for opioid withdrawal. The legal restrictions changed, allowing physicians to prescribe methadone for pain. It can be difficult, however, to get methadone dispensed at local pharmacies that aren't associated with a withdrawal clinic. While they can legally dispense methadone prescribed for pain treatment, many choose not to stock or dispense it due to abuse concerns.

It's realistic to have a pain patient get methadone from a local pharmacy if he can find one willing to dispense it.

Methadone is very complicated to dose correctly for pain. In fact, this resulted in numerous accidental overdose deaths in the early 2000s and caused methadone to fall out of favor with many pain clinics. However, some specialty clinics still prescribe methadone for chronic pain under strict guidelines and cautions. If your character is getting methadone for pain, she'll likely need regular blood tests to prove she's taking (and not selling) her pills.

Despite restricted access, methadone is heavily abused. It's purchased from drug dealers, and clinic take-home doses are stockpiled to take several all at once. Some abusers "stack" (combine) methadone with benzodiazepines, alcohol, or other opioids, like oxycodone, for a bigger high. It's also not uncommon for heroin addicts treated at methadone clinics to be on a low maintenance dosing of methadone for years while continuing to periodically abuse heroin for the addictive rush.

Methadone is often abused together with other drugs to get a bigger high.

Many chronic pain patients were left with untreated pain when opioid prescribing restrictions were instituted due to the opioid crisis and rising overdoses. Some of these patients lost their battle against their pain, resulting in suicide. Some turned to illicit street drugs. If this is your character, having her find a way to buy methadone for her pain would be realistic. Surprisingly, many drugs are easy to find and can even be purchased through social media apps. However, she's more likely to buy cheaper and readily available oxycodone pain pills. And *now* your character faces other dangers since street drugs, such as oxycodone, are increasingly tainted with fentanyl, often in lethal amounts (see "Fentanyl" in this chapter).

Ironically, methadone itself causes withdrawal when it's stopped too quickly. For example, if your main character's being treated in a methadone program for a heroin addiction and suddenly gets kidnapped, she'll suffer both methadone withdrawal *and* heroin cravings.

If you're considering having a character that's going through an opioid withdrawal program using methadone, or any of the other possible treatments, it would be important to have a medical addiction specialist review your manuscript for authenticity due to the complexity and ongoing changes in such programs as well as the behaviors of those undergoing treatment.

Slang Terms

(Since terminology and slang terms change over time, further research is highly encouraged.)

Street names

fizzies, wafer

How is it used?

In hospitals, methadone is given as an injection, tablet, or liquid. The previously orange-flavored methadone liquid has been replaced by a concentrated cherry-flavored syrup (or in some cases, unflavored). Liquids are often used at methadone treatment clinics instead of pills to reduce the risk of the pills being diverted and sold. Some clinics dispense dose wafers, however.

Methadone is most often abused as pills, powder, or liquid. Strong flavored juices help mask the bitter flavor of the powder and pills.

It's realistic for your methadone-abusing character to stockpile her take-home doses from the OTP, then take several of the doses all at once to get high. The character can also "stack" other opioids with the methadone, for example, taking oxycodone and methadone together in an attempt to get an even bigger high.

As mentioned, methadone can cause an overdose. This may be from an incorrect dose or an intentionally high dose. It can also occur accidentally by an inexperienced user who, unaware of the more subtle high that methadone causes, might take higher and higher doses in an effort to get a rush, risking an overdose.

Now you try it

> **Writing Prompt #1** Decide which of your characters has a backstory that includes treatment with methadone for an opioid addiction. How did your character originally become addicted? What drove the character into a treatment program? How has the past impacted the character's current daily life and worldview? (You'll use this background in Writing Prompt #2.)

How will my character act or feel?

If your character is using methadone to withdraw from an opioid, she'll feel fewer cravings after her treatment doses. But her withdrawal symptoms might start returning before her next dose is due. The treatment doses won't give her euphoria, but if she stockpiles doses and then takes enough to get high she'll be drowsy, lightheaded, mentally foggy, and slur her words. She'll have stomach pain, nausea, and vomiting. With a high enough methadone dose, she'll pass out and her breathing could stop. Alcohol will accelerate this risk.

Withdrawal from methadone will cause your character to suffer tremors, nausea, severe abdominal cramps, intense vomiting, severe diarrhea, hot and cold flushes, sweating, runny noses and eyes, drug cravings, insomnia, and mood changes. She won't die from methadone withdrawal, unless she develops life-threatening dehydration from the vomiting and diarrhea. She's going to feel horrible, driving a desire for more methadone. Or, she might turn to heroin.

Now you try it

> **Writing Prompt #2** Write a scene using the background from Writing Prompt #1. The character has been secretly abusing methadone. Why? How's this revealed?

How long will this drug affect my character?

When used for pain, methadone only lasts four to eight hours. For withdrawal, it can help reduce the symptoms of withdrawal from other opioids for up to twenty-four to forty-eight hours, although symptoms may start well before the next scheduled methadone dose. Withdrawal symptoms from methadone itself can start twelve to forty-eight hours after the last dose and can last one to two weeks (or more).

PUTTING IT ALL TOGETHER

> **Sample Scenario** Pat couldn't take the pain any more. He couldn't sleep. Walking hurt too much. The methadone just wasn't helping. Maybe if he took an extra pill, or two, he'd feel better. He reached for the bottle, shaking several into his palm. If this doesn't work, he'd call the doctor tomorrow. He swallowed the pills and laid back to watch a movie, waiting for his pain to fade.

Now you try it

> **Writing Prompt #3** Continue writing the scene with Pat (above). What does he feel like when those pills start working? How does this scene end?

MORPHINE

Brief History/Social Context

Morphine, named after Morpheus, the Greek god of dreams, wasn't isolated from opium poppies until the early 1800s, but its effects on pain were known as far back as 1500 BC. When the breakthrough invention of syringes in the mid-1800s allowed morphine to be injected, pain control entered a new era. Since then, morphine has had a complex history of use, abuse, and legal restrictions. From the pain management of wounded soldiers during the US Civil War to the modern-day reduction of cancer pain, morphine has been a staple of care. But the euphoria it causes has also led to a long history of abuse and, ultimately, addiction. During the Civil War, the morphine used to treat the painful wounds of soldiers was often continued long after they returned home from battle, lending to addiction. In addition, morphine was also regularly prescribed for a wide variety of ailments. As the problem of addiction grew, physicians began to reduce the amount of morphine prescribed and change the way they treated pain. But finding a drug as powerful against severe pain was challenging and morphine use continued to be a mainstay of treatment.

Morphine remains a valuable treatment today. However, unlike in the mid-1800s, morphine is unlikely to be prescribed except in certain cases of severe pain, such as from cancer or during surgery. For other painful conditions, a wide variety of other opioids, like Vicodin (hydrocodone with acetaminophen) or oxycodone have been more commonly prescribed. Even these opioids, however, are used less due to recent prescribing restrictions that were developed in response to the growing opioid overdoses in the US. Now, not only will your contemporary character not be given morphine elixir or tablets after a tonsillectomy but he'll also probably not be prescribed *any* opioid.

Does this mean your modern-day character can't struggle with a morphine addiction? Absolutely not. Morphine is still abused, although much less often due to the vast supplies of cheap and easy to obtain oxycodone, fentanyl, and heroin. But your character's grandmother with cancer may have morphine tablets at home that your character pilfers—initially to get high and eventually to avoid withdrawal. But if he keeps taking morphine, he runs the risk of an overdose that can slow his breathing down to the point of death. Or he may move on to street drugs, such as oxycodone or fentanyl, when his grandmother's supply is gone (see "Oxycodone" and "Fentanyl" in this chapter).

Morphine scenes can revolve around traditional storylines, such as a character's severe pain or a character struggling with a morphine addiction. But there are also a few unique related topics that can offer writers interesting scenarios to consider. A few of those will be discussed here, including theft of morphine from a hospital, the use of poppy seeds to control pain, and the truth about poppy seed bagels and failed urine drug screens.

Your Civil War soldier could be given a morphine elixir to use at home after his surgery, but this will not be an option for many modern-day scenarios.

Stealing morphine in a hospital is very difficult to do in the modern era. For decades, narcotics like morphine have been stored in restricted areas. In the patient bed areas in many hospitals, it's stored in robotic cabinets that require access with a security code or a fingerprint scan. The machine records each time the cabinet is opened, by whom, and what was removed. Getting morphine from these cabinets also often requires a second nurse to enter a security code as a witness regarding which narcotic was used, how much was used, and how much of the remaining drug was discarded. There are usually additional security requirements to inventory the amount of each narcotic left in the machine at the end of each shift. In some rural or small hospitals that can't afford these expensive robotic cabinets, morphine may be kept in locked drawers in the patient care unit or stored only in the hospital pharmacy. Only certain employees can access the morphine in these cases. Even inside the pharmacies, there are additional security measures for narcotics, such as morphine, to be kept inside a robotic machine or a separate locked room. Phew! That's a *lot* of security for your character to overcome.

Don't have your antagonist easily reach into a drawer and steal morphine in a hospital.

So, what's a plausible way for your character to steal morphine in a hospital? In the patient care areas of a hospital, those robotic cabinets are often kept in a separate locked room. There have been cases of nurses entering the room and taking a morphine vial out of the robotic cabinet. When the computer prompts for the witness security code, a savvy nurse may enter the numbers borrowed from another nurse that was too overwhelmed with a sick patient to come to the machine. Are nurses supposed to give out their codes? No. But overworked, overwhelmed nurses sometimes have. Then, it only takes a few minutes for your character to pop the plastic cap off of the vial, pull all the morphine out with a syringe, refill the vial with sterile water, and replace it into the machine. An experienced nurse can do this entire process in under a minute. The nurse can then enter a code to cancel the dose originally requested from the machine. With a full syringe of morphine in the pocket of her scrubs, she can leave the room unnoticed.

Does this sound almost *too* easy for your character? There's a catch. There's a big chance the nurse will get caught. How? Other nurses or doctors can become suspicious from important clues left behind. Remember that little plastic protective cap that was popped off? That would be obviously missing. Although, those do pop off easily enough that the clue might be missed. But there will be a needle hole, albeit a small one, in the rubber stopper on the morphine vial. An astute nurse will notice and suspect the vial has been used. But if the puncture mark is tiny enough and the vial is full of liquid, the theft might still go unnoticed by a busy nurse. So, what *will* make people suspicious? When a patient's agonizing pain doesn't improve after a couple of doses of "morphine" from *that* vial, but really improves after a dose from a *different* vial, the nurses will begin to realize there's a problem.

How will your character plausibly be caught? Remember, that robotic cabinet keeps track of everyone entering that machine. A manager will likely compare a report from the machine to the nurses working that day and begin an investigation, narrowing down the suspects.

A tiny puncture or two in a vial stopper can be the first clue of drug tampering.

What about the possibility of a character stealing morphine right out of those infusion bags hanging by a patient's hospital bedside? Again, rather difficult. Historically, morphine bags were hung on a pole next to a patient, with a pump that was programmed to give the right dose. *Anyone* could have slipped a syringe into the bag to steal morphine (and some people did). But in recent decades, those bags have become more secure to keep people from stealing the morphine. Now, generally those bags must either be locked inside a plastic protective shell or be within view of the nurses. So, a movie scene where a visitor goes into a patient's private room, closes the door, then shoves a syringe into the morphine bag to steal some for himself may work in a 1980s setting, but not in a contemporary storyline. There may be some exceptions, but don't count on that for your scene.

You may be surprised to know that not only are those morphine bags locked up tightly, but the *program* on the pump is also locked. A security code is usually needed to change the morphine dose. Why? Because there have been unfortunate cases of the dose on the pump being altered by parents, visitors, or even the patient. In some cases, the patient has died of an overdose. Even on special pumps called "patient-controlled analgesia," which allow the patient to push a button for more morphine, the programs are locked. The doctor decides the maximum number of extra doses to allow, and the pump won't give any after that, no matter how many times the button is pushed. And the pump will record every time the button is pushed. While this helps the doctor determine if he's giving the patient enough pain medicine, it can also help identify attempted unscrupulous acts by a visitor.

A villain may try to tamper with a morphine infusion, but it can be difficult in contemporary storylines.

Despite all the safeguards, narcotics such as morphine are stolen and abused by a small number of healthcare professionals. Recent headlines of numerous fentanyl vials stolen and replaced with saline show that it can be done. If you are looking for additional ways to depict your character getting around hospital safeguards, a hospital nurse or pharmacist would make an excellent critique partner to help you craft a believable scenario.

If you're looking for a more natural opioid for your character to use, morphine is still a great option. Did you know that opium poppy seeds are naturally coated in a layer of morphine? Washing the seeds removes most (but not all) of the morphine, but illicit markets sell unwashed seeds. These seeds have become popular to brew into teas to treat pain, calm opiate withdrawal symptoms, or even to get high.

But these innocent looking seeds can also cause trouble for your protagonist. If he regularly uses morphine-coated seeds, he can develop a tolerance, meaning he'll need increasing doses to control his pain or get his high. And if he stops taking them, he'll suffer morphine withdrawal symptoms. Believe it or not, since poppy seed production is not regulated, the character could overdose from an unexpectedly potent batch. In fact, after the 2016 death of a college student who overdosed on seeds he purchased online the Food and Drug Administration (FDA) banned the sales of unwashed poppy seeds. But don't worry, your character can still realistically get the seeds. The unwashed seeds are *still* for sale online—the websites just no longer advertise the morphine content and don't identify them as unwashed.

Unwashed poppy seeds could lead to a morphine overdose in your character.

Don't get these morphine poppy seeds confused with everyday "baking" poppy seeds, however, such as those used to make poppy seed bagels. Baking seeds are specifically grown to contain low morphine concentrations and are washed before selling to remove the morphine residue. It's important to know these seeds still do contain *some* morphine, though. So, *is* it realistic for a character to fail a urine drug screen because of that little bit of morphine from eating a poppy seed bagel? The answer is yes. Within thirty minutes of eating a bagel topped with a generous amount of poppy seeds, urine can have enough morphine to be detected on a drug screen. It can even be detected up to one to two days after eating that bagel. If your story takes place before 1998, eating just *one* poppy seed bagel could believably set your character up to fail a drug screen. To get rid of the problem of tests being failed due to a common food, the detection limits on the lab tests were adjusted in 1998. So, in a scene set after this adjustment your character is *less likely* to fail the screen after eating that single bagel. However, reports of failed tests from people eating more than one bagel (or a single bagel with a very generous amount of poppy seeds) do continue. Despite the lab changes, bagels still pose a risk to your character. With the required procedures and legalities regarding failed urine drug screens constantly changing, have a local lab technician beta read your draft to assure believability.

Your modern-day character likely won't fail a urine drug screen from eating a single poppy seed bagel, but if he eats a couple . . . he might.

Slang Terms

(Since terminology and slang terms change over time, further research is highly encouraged.)

Street names

dreamer, M, Miss Emma, monkey, Mr. Blue, MS, white stuff

Weaving the Plot

How is it used?

Medical morphine is available as injections, infusions, tablets (short acting, long acting, and sublingual), and oral syrup. Abusers may inject (slam) morphine, snort morphine powder, or dissolve the crushed, bitter pills in tea. The regular morphine tablets may be crushed to snort, but many users complain of the slower, less intense high and prefer to boof (insert rectally) diluted tablets. Many longer-acting morphine pill formulations use new technology to keep abusers from being able to inject or snort them. For example, some tablets have been designed to turn into a gel when crushed or diluted. Savvy users, however, know how to make special salted dilutions or cook the morphine to avoid the gel formation stage.

Now you try it

> **Writing Prompt #1** Write a scene where one of your characters decides to make poppy seed tea to help with back pain. How did the character find out about them and get them? (You'll continue this scene in Writing Prompt #2.)

How will my character act or feel?

Like other opiates, morphine will help your character's pain decrease, may make him feel drowsy, and create a pleasant lightheadedness. When used to get high, these effects are magnified. Injected or boofed, morphine will cause a rapid high. Your character will not be able to think clearly, will stagger, and will slur his words. If he's been snorting morphine, he may have crusty, bleeding sores around his nose. For an interesting twist, some people experience hallucinations, such as seeing spiders crawling on the wall, with normal doses of opioids such as morphine.

Chronic morphine will cause your protagonist to need higher and higher doses to get the same euphoria. This can set the stage for an overdose with dangerously slow breathing, severe mental confusion, clammy cool skin, a slow heart rate, blue lips and fingertips (from low oxygen). Your character may have a seizure that causes foam to drip from his mouth as his body convulses. Finally, his breathing could slow to a stop. If he gets a dose of naloxone antidote in time (see "A Word about Antidotes" in chapter 3), he may survive. Even with the emergency antidote, if his breathing isn't restarted quickly enough, brain damage can leave him with permanent disabilities (see the appendix). If your character tries to stop taking morphine, he'll suffer withdrawal symptoms. He'll feel like he has the flu, with severe muscle aches, sneezing, a runny nose, insomnia, nausea, vomiting, and potentially severe diarrhea. He'll also be yawning frequently. Will your character survive withdrawal? Yes, unless his vomiting and diarrhea lead to life-threatening dehydration.

Morphine can make a character believe he sees spiders on the wall.

Injecting morphine can leave telltale needle marks (track marks) along his skin, such as on his forearm or the crook of his elbow, although they can be anywhere that he's injected his morphine. The track marks can be irritated or infected. If he's shared needles with other drug abusers, he's at risk for certain diseases, such as hepatitis or HIV.

Now you try it

> **Writing Prompt #2** Write a scene using your character from Writing Prompt #1. The poppy seed tea worked great for the first couple of weeks, but now it's taking a lot more seeds in the tea to control the pain. Unfortunately, your character can't afford more seeds right now. What is the character's day like?

How long will this drug affect my character?

Pain control from injecting morphine can begin within a few minutes (three to five). The high, however, begins within a minute. Snorting morphine causes a less intense euphoria in about five minutes. Boofing can have a five-minute delay to the high, but it's more intense than from snorting. A morphine high can last about an hour, while the sedation and drowsiness can last for three to four hours. Unfortunately, pain control may only last as little as two hours, making it tempting to take more too soon. There are also many long-acting morphine products that last twelve to twenty-four hours.

PUTTING IT ALL TOGETHER

> **Sample Scenario #1** A. J. crushes the pill, hoping Grandma won't notice it's missing. He quickly snorts it, then wipes the powder from his nose. Leaning back onto his pillows with his phone, he flicks past videos, waiting for the buzzy high he knows is on the way.

Now you try it

> **Writing Prompt #3** Choose one of your own characters to have a morphine addiction. How did the habit begin? Why? How does the addiction impact your character's life?

Opium

Brief History/Social Context

Opium brings the possibilities of scenes of injured Civil War soldiers addicted to pain medicine or housewives of the late 1800s frequenting opium dens. Opium is a powerful pain medication that's harvested from the milky-white latex in the unripened seed pods harvested from the poppy plant, *Papaver somniferum*. Once dried, the highest quality opium is brown and sticky. Importantly, opium is the source of all other opiate drugs. Some, like morphine or codeine, are extracted right from opium, but many others, like heroin, oxycodone, or fentanyl, must be made by a chemical conversion of opium. The opium plants used to make illicit street drugs, such as heroin, are grown in a number of countries throughout the world. But all the opium used to make medications must be imported from specially designated countries to regulate its consistency since cultivation is illegal in the US. So while opium harvested from poppy fields in Mexico may work for a story, it will not be realistic to have your opium-growing antagonist living on a farm in Iowa.

The medicinal use of opium dates back to at least 3400 BC. It was hailed as a remedy by Greek and Roman physicians for pain, intestinal ailments, and insomnia. It's even still used as a medicinal treatment today.

Unfortunately, opium also has a long history of abuse and addiction. The high from opium causes an addictive, euphoric "rush," with a pleasurable warmth, but it can also cause deadly overdoses. Taking too much opium can cause your character's breathing to become dangerously slow (or completely stop). He can suffer a seizure, a loss of consciousness, lapse into a coma, and die.

After just a few opium doses, the euphoric rush can tempt your character to want more.

Despite the risks, opium addiction grew rapidly in the US through a combination of opium dens in the mid-1800s, treatment of wounded soldiers during the Civil War, and recreational use. During this time period in history, your character could have smoked, injected, or swallowed opium to get high. He might have smoked it at one of the many popular opium dens in the US that led to widespread addiction. He could have purchased "laudanum," an opium tincture, from a pharmacist to treat his wife's stomach ailment. Or he could have returned from war and become addicted to opium from ongoing treatment of his painful wounds.

Addiction became such a problem in the US that the Opium Poppy Control Act of 1942 was passed to restrict the growth and use of opium to medical treatment. The unintended consequence of this was that opium users simply shifted to taking heroin, which was easier to get. Interestingly, a government crackdown on heroin in 1960 caused a new surge of opium use.

Opium abuse has decreased in the US over many decades, replaced initially by heroin and most recently by the skyrocketing abuse of oxycodone and fentanyl. But opium is still smoked and abused in the US today. Even as recently as 2022, an illegal shipment of opium pods was confiscated in the US. These pods can be used to extract opium or the residue inside them can be scraped to smoke. So, while it isn't as popular as many other drugs of abuse, there continue to be pockets of opium users that can believably be woven into your plot or your protagonist's backstory.

In a 1960s setting, a government crackdown may make your heroin-using character turn to opium for his high.

Opium use brings visions of smoke-filled opium dens. But both historical and contemporary fiction authors can make use of two unique opium products that pose serious risks when used incorrectly and have led to numerous fatalities. One product is paregoric elixir, a longstanding treatment for stomach ailments and diarrhea. This noxious-smelling mixture of opium, camphor, and about 40 percent alcohol could be purchased until the 1960s in pharmacies without a prescription in many states. This made paregoric an easy alternative high for heroin users, but because it was too foul to drink, they injected it. But don't have your character pull paregoric directly into a syringe from the bottle: the paregoric had to be boiled first to remove the camphor (which can cause seizures) before it was injected. By the 1960s, paregoric was finally restricted to requiring a prescription in the US to curb abuse.

Paregoric could have been used to help calm drug withdrawal in your character's newborn baby.

Paregoric elixir is still prescribed today for diarrhea. It continues to contain ingredients that make the taste and odor extremely foul. So, it isn't likely that a character would swig back lots of paregoric for an opium high, at least not without vomiting much of it and feeling terrible afterward. As recently as the early 2000s, paregoric was also used to treat newborns suffering narcotic withdrawal. However, because of the risk of seizures from the camphor, doctors switched to treating the withdrawal with morphine instead.

Another useful medication with potentially lethal risks is tincture of opium (historically called laudanum). From its sleepy euphoria to its ability to calm intestinal ailments, such as diarrhea, tincture of opium has a long history of use and abuse. What's the danger? Tincture of opium has *twenty-five times more opium* than paregoric. Because it's so concentrated, it must be diluted before taking a dose. Unfortunately, the accidental use of undiluted tincture of opium has led to multiple fatalities. It's also realistic for a person to have both tincture of opium and paregoric at home. A simple measurement error—taking a teaspoonful of the tincture instead of paregoric—will spin a scene into a new direction.

In the world of medicine, countless cases of name confusion between drugs have led to many overdoses, and paregoric and tincture of opium are no different. And while these cases are sad, they lend themselves to simple plot twists. Paregoric (also called "diluted tincture of opium") gets confused with tincture of opium (also called "deodorized tincture of opium"). Sound confusing? It gets even *more* complicated—the abbreviation "DTO" has often been used by doctors to prescribe both of these medicines. Not surprisingly, this has led to tragedies. If one of your characters is given tincture of opium, instead of paregoric, he'll get twenty-five times the amount of opium intended, suffer overdose symptoms, and possibly die. This problem decreased as doctors began using electronic prescriptions because the computers would not allow the abbreviations. But this concept could easily be incorporated into stories plotted during the era of hand-written prescriptions.

Confusion surrounding paregoric and tincture of opium could put your character in peril.

Would you be surprised that something as innocent as poppy seeds could lead to a plot twist? Not only are the seed pods from the *Papaver somniferum* plants filled with opium resin but the little seeds inside the pods are coated in a substance that's relatively high in morphine. Washing the seeds removes most of the morphine, but unwashed seeds are popular to make into tea to treat pain, reduce opiate withdrawal symptoms, or just to get high (see "Morphine" in this chapter).

Slang Terms

(Since terminology and slang terms change over time, further research is highly encouraged.)

Street names

Auntie Emma, big O, Chinese molasses, dopium, joy plant, midnight oil, Opie

Other terms

- Black: opium combined with marijuana and methamphetamine.
- Blue Velvet: a combination of opium from boiled paregoric and the antihistamine tripelennamine hydrochloride, which creates a blue liquid to inject.
- Budda: opium combined with marijuana.

Weaving the Plot

How is it used?

Both paregoric and tincture of opium are oral liquids. While paregoric is dosed by the teaspoonful, tincture of opium is an extremely concentrated liquid that must be diluted before use to avoid a twenty-five-fold deadly overdose. Until about 1960, paregoric was injected by abusers for the opium high, after boiling off the camphor (to avoid seizures) and straining the cooled liquid through a cotton ball. Street opium, a brownish powder, is smoked, injected, or swallowed. Unwashed poppy seeds can be boiled to make tea. The white coating on poppy seed pods can be wiped onto a cigarette or blunt (marijuana cigarette) to smoke. Street opium is also smoked using many of the same devices used for marijuana (see "Marijuana" in chapter 12).

Now you try it

> **Writing Prompt #1** Develop a scene for one of your characters whose friend offers some "special" weed to smoke that's mixed with opium. What would your character do in this situation? (You'll continue this scene in Writing Prompt #2.)

How will my character act or feel?

Oral paregoric has such a noxious taste and odor that your character may vomit from the dose. But if enough paregoric stays in his stomach, his diarrhea or intestinal cramps will calm down. Tincture of opium will cause a slight drowsiness and relaxation at regular doses. If your character smokes or injects opium, he'll experience an intense rush (similar to heroin), followed by extreme relaxation and drowsiness. The feeling has been described as being wrapped in a warm blanket. A poppy seed tea will give this calm, relaxed feeling, as well, but without the rush. Your character's world will drift slowly by. He might vomit, be drowsy, feel dizzy, have trouble concentrating, and have a dry mouth. After the high is gone (after the "come down"), he'll feel hungover.

Is the character injecting opium? His injection sites can become infected, leaving angry red sores. Or he might contract a disease, such as hepatitis or HIV, from sharing needles with others.

With overdoses, opium causes dangerously slow (or completely stopped) breathing. Without the emergency antidote, naloxone, your character could die (see "A Word about Antidotes" in chapter 3). Even with rapid medical care, if his breathing isn't restarted quickly enough, your character can suffer brain damage with a wide range of permanent disabilities (see the appendix). Keep in mind that naloxone wasn't available until the 1970s, so don't plan on this lifesaving drug for your Civil War hero or a character injecting too much paregoric in a story set in the 1950s.

Withdrawal from opium, like other opioids, can feel like a very bad case of the flu, complete with severe body aches, profuse cold sweats, light-sensitive eyes, a dripping nose, nausea, vomiting, and diarrhea. He'll also be frequently yawning. Without enough fluids, he can develop life-threatening dehydration.

Now you try it

> **Writing Prompt #2** Continue the scene from Writing Prompt #1. Your character gives into peer pressure and decides to take a few hits of the opium-laced weed. How does the character feel? What's the experience like? How does the scene end?

How long will this drug affect my character?

Diarrhea and intestinal cramps can be calmed in fifteen to twenty minutes. The rapid euphoric rush from smoking heroin begins within seconds. The less intense high from swallowing opium can take about twenty to thirty minutes to be felt. The effects from opium are more pronounced in the first hour and slowly decrease over about four hours.

Sample Scenario "Here." The nurse holds the spoon for the trembling old woman. "This will help with the diarrhea."

The woman swallows the liquid and smiles. "Oh, my. That *other* nurse gives me the most awful tasting medicine. This is so much better!"

"Good!" the nurse says, tucking the blankets around the frail woman. "Now, take a good nap."

The nurse relaxes into an armchair, opens a book, and begins reading. Soon her eyes flutter closed. When she finally wakes, she gently shakes the sleeping woman. "Like to try a bit of soup now?"

Now you try it

Writing Prompt #3 Continue writing the scene above with a twist: there are two medicine bottles on the bedside table—the one the nurse gave the spoonful from and a bottle of paregoric. How does the scene progress?

OXYCODONE

Brief History/Social Context

Oxycodone, better known as "oxy," is an opioid pain drug that's been around since the early 1900s and prescribed for pain since the 1940s. Prescribing increased in the 1960s with the availability of Percodan, which combined oxycodone with aspirin. By the 1970s, oxycodone was combined with acetaminophen in Percocet tablets (see "A Note of Caution: Using Brand Names" in chapter 1). Oxycodone (in any form) has a long history of abuse for the strong euphoria it causes. To combat rampant abuse, in the mid-1990s manufacturers developed a special formulation of oxycodone, called OxyContin, a twelve-hour slow-releasing pill offering no euphoria. But it was quickly discovered that chewing or snorting crushed OxyContin *did* give a potent high by releasing all twelve hours of the drug at once and it soon became known as hillbilly heroin. Various other special formulations have been

> **Your character might resort to heroin use when his oxycodone tablets turn to gel when he crushes them.**

developed, including one that turns the tablet into a gel if it's crushed, making it unusable. These also worked to temporarily decrease abuse. However, many frustrated oxycodone abusers turned to heroin instead. Eventually, ways to get around the abuse deterrents were discovered and oxycodone abuse has continued ever since.

Overprescribing made it easier to find oxycodone to feed an addiction.

Over the last several years, oxycodone has gained true notoriety as part of the escalating overdoses and deaths during the opioid crisis. This crisis was, in part, initially fueled by the overprescribing of opioid pills, like oxycodone, starting in the 1990s. This caused an oversupply of pain pills that could be stolen, abused, or sold.

In response to the crisis, starting in about 2017 opioid prescribing became progressively restricted to decrease opioid use and abuse. The unintended consequences of this, however, was an increase in the black market demand for pills like oxycodone. Drug traffickers exploited this demand by flooding the market with cheap counterfeit oxycodone tablets made to look like brand name pills. These "Mexican oxy" pills are grayish blue, stamped with an "M" on one side and a "30" on the other. The large supply of these pills has made them cheap and easy to buy. They can even be found for sale on social media apps.

Poorly treated pain could cause your protagonist to seek out street oxycodone.

And it's not just people looking to get high from oxycodone that are seeking out street oxy. The rapid rollout of opioid prescribing restrictions left some chronic pain patients with debilitating pain. Some of these people committed suicide. Some turned to street drugs.

Many of the counterfeit pain pills, however, contain fentanyl that's added by drug traffickers to boost the high. Unfortunately, selling the pills is more important to the traffickers than mixing them carefully. So while some of the pills contain very little fentanyl, many of them contain lethal amounts.

What does all this mean for your story? Oxycodone offers you scenarios dating back to the 1960s, from a character suffering serious pain after surgery to one that's stealing her mom's pain pills to get high or even sell at school. It also offers an unexpected plot twist—your character getting high on oxy

A character buying illicit oxy pills could die of a fentanyl overdose.

could actually die of a *fentanyl* overdose. In fact, if your story is set in the early 2020s, it's much more realistic to have your character overdose on a fentanyl-tainted pill than from prescription oxycodone (see "Fentanyl" in this chapter).

Slang Terms

(Since terminology and slang terms change over time, further research is highly encouraged.)

Street names

hillbilly heroin, kicker, Mexican oxy, OCs, ox, oxy, perc (for Percocet), roxy (for Roxicet)

Weaving the Plot

How is it used?

Oxycodone and oxy combination medicines are available as pills. If a character's abusing oxycodone, he may swallow the pills or crush them into a powder to either snort, mix into a drink, or dilute to inject. Crushed powder can also be heated on bits of foil to inhale the fumes. The twelve-hour extended-release pills are crushed to snort or inject for the dramatic high despite the risk of death. Some formulations are designed to turn into gels when crushed to hamper abuse, which can make for a humorous scene. Or if your character is savvy, she might cook the pill before crushing it to get around the gel deterrent or just swallow the pill whole.

Now you try it

> **Writing Prompt #1** Pick one of your own characters to sneak oxycodone from someone's medicine cabinet. After several of the pills are swallowed, the rest are pocketed for later. Whose pills are they? What's the motivation to do this? (You'll continue this scene in Writing Prompt #2.)

How will my character act or feel?

Oxycodone causes a light-headed high, relaxation, drowsiness, and difficulty thinking clearly. With a high dose, your character should experience a euphoria, extreme drowsiness, weakness, and severe confusion. With an overdose, she'll pass out and her breathing will become dangerously slow. Without enough oxygen, her lips may turn bluish. If she has a seizure, she could collapse to the floor with convulsions and foam might drip from her mouth. And her breathing could completely stop. Without the emergency antidote naloxone, your character will not make it to the next scene. Even with naloxone, if her breathing isn't restored to a safe level soon enough, brain damage can leave her with permanent disabilities (see the appendix).

Overdoses of combination oxycodone pills create other dangers. In addition to the opioid overdose symptoms, the high dose of acetaminophen can lead to severe liver damage and a slow, painful death. With aspirin containing pills, toxic levels can cause numerous symptoms, including seizures, dangerous heart rhythms, brain damage, and death. In both of these cases, your character is in serious peril even after the naloxone antidote and needs emergency medical care. Because of the complexity of these overdoses, if you're using one of these combination drugs in your scenario, further research into acetaminophen or aspirin toxicity is recommended.

If the character injects oxy, in addition to sores at her injection sites, she risks contracting hepatitis or HIV from sharing needles, even once, with an infected user.

Now you try it

> **Writing Prompt #2** Your character from Writing Prompt #1 is found unconscious on the floor. Who finds your character? How does the scene unfold? Can you end this scene in a page-turner?

How long will the drug affect my character?

Sedation (and with higher doses, a strong euphoria) starts in about fifteen to thirty minutes and can last about two hours with regular tablets. Pain control can last two to four hours. However, snorting these quick-acting pills can cause a rapid high within a few seconds, lasting only about an hour. With the twelve-hour pills the slow drug release causes only subtle sedation without the rapid high. Pain control from these may last as long as twelve hours.

Overdose symptoms from oxycodone short-acting or combination tablets can start within fifteen to thirty minutes, depending on how it's taken. If a *nonlethal* overdose was taken, the character may act very drunk and clumsy, pass out, and remain unconscious for several hours. As long as her breathing or heart rate is not impacted, she'll be alright when the drug wears off, although she may still be very groggy. But if her breathing has slowed or stopped, she'll need an emergency dose of the antidote naloxone to avoid dying (see chapter 3). When the slow-release pills are swallowed whole, a steady amount of oxycodone is released for up to twelve hours. Crushing and snorting these pills will rapidly cause euphoria within five to ten minutes. Swallowed in an overdose, however, these long-acting pills will continue to release oxycodone long after a naloxone antidote has been given. Your character will be hit with another wave (or several) of overdose symptoms when the naloxone wears off. She'll need regular antidote doses over several hours until the threat of death has passed.

See all the possible plot twists here?

PUTTING IT ALL TOGETHER

Sample Scenario Alex leans back heavily against the couch, fumbling with the remote. His eyelids droop. Wasn't he going to watch something? It doesn't matter. He feels *so* good. His eyes drift to the table and he laughs. Why not? He leans in, pinching one side of his nose and snorts his last line of oxy. He lets the bitterness drip down his throat and watches the room swirl.

Now you try it

Writing Prompt #3 Write a scene involving a character whose severe pain has been treated with oxycodone ever since a serious car accident a year ago. Now, the doctor won't prescribe more pills for fear of addiction. But the pain is coming back. And it's bad. There's a rumor that a guy has pain pills for sale down near the gas station. What does your character decide to do? What happens next?

14

SEDATIVES

Sedatives can offer a wide variety of dramatic scenes, from patients sedated in asylums to lethal plot twists. What many people call "sedatives" are technically broken into two kinds of drugs: hypnotics that induce sleep and sedatives that create calm and drowsiness. In general, these drugs are used for a variety of conditions, including insomnia (sleeping pills), anxiety, surgical sedation, and even seizures. For the purposes of this chapter, the word *sedatives* will be generically used to mean both sedatives and hypnotics.

There are so many sedatives to consider throughout history that it would be impossible to cover them all. This chapter will focus on a few well-known sedatives that offer interesting options for both historical fiction and modern-era storylines. Key similarities and differences, uses, and important historical ramifications to consider for plotting will be included. Importantly, the information will not only clarify how to create believable scenes using sedatives but also what should be avoided. These principles can be applied to many other sedatives or to "author-inspired" sedative-type drugs.

What sedatives are discussed here? Chloroform, chloral hydrate, bromides, barbiturates, benzodiazepines, "z-drugs," "truth serum," and even melatonin.

Brief History/Social Context

Remember those dramatic movie scenes where a chloroform-saturated rag held over a character's face makes her instantly go limp and stay unconscious long after the rag is gone? Actually, this scene is unrealistic. Chloroform takes several minutes to knock someone out, even with that rag fully covering the face. And soon after the rag is removed, the person will start to arouse. A more honest scene would have the poor character struggling for several minutes against the kidnapper as the chloroform slowly takes effect. Then the kidnapper will have to figure out how to keep that drug-soaked rag in place and keep the victim unconscious without (and this is key) the chloroform

It's not realistic to have chloroform knock out a character within seconds.

killing her. Phew! While the bad guy's fumbling with duct tape and the rag, the viewers are probably turning off the show.

The process of picking the right sedative for your scene should include making sure it actually works the way you need it to. And the historical setting of the story will also be a big factor in credibility. The availability, trends, and popularity of sedatives have changed dramatically as the risks of some drugs came to light and new drugs were discovered.

Chloral Hydrate

Chloral hydrate was a popular sedative and anti-seizure treatment in the late-nineteenth and early-twentieth centuries. However, it fell into disfavor because of serious side effects, such as dangerously slowed breathing, that lead to death. In addition, once finally awake after a dose, some patients experienced an unexpected second wave of sedation—with some of them dying. Despite this, chloral hydrate continued to be prescribed until it was withdrawn from the market in 2012. For a while, reports of chloral hydrate–related deaths decreased. But when scattered reports of additional deaths occurred, it was discovered that chloral hydrate use had resumed. Driven in part by the cheap cost of chloral hydrate, compounding pharmacies had begun making it for local hospitals and dentists. However, because of legal implications and the potential dangers, chloral hydrate has largely been replaced by safer alternatives.

Bromides

The strong sedative effects of bromides were widely used in the late 1800s to treat seizures and sedate combative and psychotic patients in asylums. Bromides caused difficulty thinking, confusion, and sluggishness. High doses were used to induce the "bromide sleep," or the "sleep cure," to treat mania and certain addictions. If your patient was given the sleep cure, she would have been completely unconscious for about five to nine *days* straight, requiring care twenty-four hours a day. This would be followed by a slow regaining of her mental and physical functions over a couple of weeks. Unfortunately, bromides also caused hallucinations and delirium. Your character might have been institutionalized for days to weeks

Bromides can cause hallucinations and delirium lasting days to weeks in your character.

waiting for her symptoms to subside. Not surprisingly, bromides were eventually phased out of use, making way for the use of barbiturates, like phenobarbital, by the early to mid-1900s.

Barbiturates

Barbiturates were first used in the early 1900s to treat seizures and, like bromides, were used for sleep cures. The earliest barbiturate was known as barbital (Veronal), followed soon after by phenobarbital, which is still used today, along with many others to treat mania, seizures, and insomnia. The barbiturate thiopental was trialed as a surgical anesthetic after the bombing of Pearl Harbor due to a shortage of anesthetic gas. This quick-acting barbiturate caused a loss of consciousness within twenty seconds. Unfortunately, a lack of experience with safe dosing resulted in a number of deaths. As the drug became better understood, thiopental was eventually adopted as a mainstream surgical anesthetic. However, the inclusion of sodium thiopental as one of the components of the lethal injection used during capital punishment led to controversy, and the drug was withdrawn from the market in 2011.

Thiopental, and its close cousin amobarbital, are also known as the "truth serums" used in psychoanalysis, some real-life interrogations, and woven into many fictional stories. But will truth serum *really* work on your character? Well, yes and no. At low doses, these drugs cause a quick "hypnotic" effect and a loss of inhibition, leaving your character more willing to talk. Does that mean your character will be truthful? Not necessarily. But these drugs do make it harder to lie since struggling against the mental cloudiness they cause to create false information takes a lot of concentration. It would take a very strong-willed character to lie. If you've developed your heroine well, her triumph over the truth serum effects will be believable.

However, your character might actually lie without even trying while under the effects of truth serum. How? Well, it turns out these truth serums have another effect: they increase suggestibility. This can make your character give the answer she thinks the interrogator *wants* to hear. Don't think this is a realistic plot line? These suggestibility effects have not only resulted in false confessions of guilt, but false "repressed childhood memories" that "resurfaced" during interviews using thiopental or amobarbital have led to lawsuits and devastated lives.

While these real incidents are unfortunate, writers can take advantage of this suggestibility effect to toss a twist into a story. *Now,* after a "therapy session," your character really *can* believe she witnessed a murder . . . or maybe thinks *she* was the killer. But your readers know the truth: it was her therapist.

Your character can falsely confess to a murder in an interview after taking "truth serum."

Are there other drugs that can be believably used in a truth serum scene? Benzodiazepines can cause similar hypnotic effects with some amnesia, but few work as quickly and intensely as thiopental or amobarbital. If you specifically refer to thiopental (or sodium pentothal) in your scene, the storyline should take place between the early 1930s and 2011.

If it takes place after that, consider referring to amobarbital or, better yet, a fictional truth serum that causes the general symptoms seen with these drugs. Veronica Roth did this well in her novel *Insurgent*, in which a fictional truth serum was given to Four and Tris, who struggled against the effects but finally succumbed. During the struggle, Tris began to believe that whatever the truth serum made her say *must* be true, causing her to question herself. Imagine taking that premise further in your story to weave a web of self-doubt and deceit.

"Truth serum" will make your character more willing to talk, but won't force her to tell the truth.

Mass prescribing of barbiturates by the mid-1900s contributed to a growing problem of addiction and abuse. By the early 1960s, there were an estimated 250,000 barbiturate addicts in the US. Deaths from barbiturate overdoses (accidental and intentional) were widely reported, the most famous of which include Marilyn Monroe and Judy Garland. High doses of barbiturates can cause breathing to slow down to the point of death—and there is no antidote. Combined with alcohol or opiates, death can be rapid. And accidental overdoses with barbiturates can easily occur in even your most innocent character. For example, a phenomenon called "automatism" can cause your character to take a second dose of her bedtime phenobarbital after forgetting that she took a dose already. In fact, this could happen several times in the same evening. A single extra dose might just put your character into a deep sleep, but what if she retook that dose a couple of times before heading to bed? And if she also lost track of how many nightcaps of brandy she'd already sipped, she could be in great danger. Writing a crime thriller or a

Mental confusion from barbiturates can make your character forget she took her dose, so she may take it again . . . a few times.

murder mystery? What if your antagonist helps your character "remember" her forgotten sleeping pill . . . a few times?

Eventually, because of the risks, barbiturates began to be replaced by benzodiazepines in the mid- to late-1950s to treat insomnia and anxiety. However, they continue to be very useful even today for treating seizures.

Benzodiazepines

Benzodiazepines ("benzos") replaced barbiturates in the 1960s for the treatment of anxiety, insomnia, and panic attacks due to better safety, since it takes a very high benzo dose to cause a person's breathing to stop unless they're taken together with alcohol or another sedative. There's also an antidote, flumazenil, for benzodiazepines (see "A Word about Antidotes" in chapter 3). "Safer" doesn't mean safe, however, and benzos can wreak plenty of havoc on your characters, from addiction to potentially deadly withdrawal.

With so many benzodiazepines becoming available over the years, how can you decide which is appropriate for your story? Avoiding specific drug names, and blending the general effects of benzos into your character's actions will always work, as long as they had historically been invented. But if you're considering being more specific, here are a few drugs matched to a general timeline: chlordiazepoxide (Librium) in the early 1960s, diazepam (Valium) in the 1960s–1970s, and alprazolam (Xanax) starting in the 1980s to the present (see "A Note of Caution: Using Brand Names" in chapter 1).

Need your character to forget part of a scene? Benzos cause short-term amnesia. Medically this is valuable to keep patients from remembering certain uncomfortable procedures or treatments. If you don't remember much about a colonoscopy, it could be from benzodiazepine sedation. The drug kept you relaxed and sleepy. It also made you forget most of what happened during the procedure. That same effect can make your character forget an entire conversation after taking her sleeping pill. Or her day can go from bad to worse when she forgets she already took that pill and takes it again. Now, dazed and unsteady on her feet, as she shuffles off to bed she falls, fracturing her hip. On a more sinister note, due to the effects of memory loss and sedation, benzos fit into date-rape scenarios (see "Club Drugs" in chapter 9).

Amnesia from a benzodiazepine offers an interesting twist.

Benzodiazepines are highly addictive, in part due to their rapid high. For contemporary plots, alprazolam (Xanax) is a well-known, popularly abused benzo. Your character might start by stealing a few of her mom's sleeping pills and end up turning to street supplies to maintain her new habit. But she won't have any trouble finding someone selling "z-bars" or "xanies." In fact, she could believably order them through a social media app, where an entire subculture using emojis and code to sell illicit drugs has been developed. But *now* your character may accidentally die since street xanies have increasingly been laced with potentially lethal amounts of fentanyl (see "Fentanyl" in chapter 13).

Z-drugs

Since the 1990s, "z-drugs" (or "z-hypnotics") have been used to treat insomnia. The nickname comes from the fact that these drugs all have the letter *z* in their name, such as zolpidem (Ambien). While they have many similarities to benzos, z-drugs cause a very unique and potentially dangerous effect: some patients perform complex tasks while *still asleep* after taking their dose.

After taking a z-drug, your character could drive the car while asleep.

These are the scenes where a character can actually be asleep while they cook a meal, drive a car, or walk off of a bridge. Assuming your character survives to the end of the scene, it's realistic for her to have no memory of what happened. But these scary effects last only a few hours. It's not believable to have your character still chasing after someone that has been "sleep-driving" since the previous night.

Like benzodiazepines, z-drugs are abused and can lead to addiction or the risk of a fentanyl overdose from counterfeit pills, offering other troubles for your character.

Melatonin

Think twice before using melatonin, the newest popular sleeping pill, in a deadly scene. Melatonin is a natural hormone made in your brain when it gets dark outside, helping to regulate the day-night cycle in your body. While it isn't a true sedative, the release of melatonin in the brain helps people fall asleep more easily. Because melatonin pills are nonaddictive and don't require a prescription in the US, they are widely used as a "natural" sleep aid. Melatonin is also used by night workers to help with daytime sleep, travelers to combat jet lag, and people who are blind to help normalize sleep patterns.

There aren't enough good studies to compare how well melatonin pills work compared to the natural hormone in the brain. But, while these pills may believably lull your protagonist to sleep, they definitely should not be used in a lethal sleeping pill scenario. High melatonin doses can leave your

sleepy character with a headache and nausea but death is extremely rare, especially in
adults. With children, most melatonin overdoses usually cause few (or no) symptoms,
but there have, unfortunately, been some
hospitalizations and deaths. These serious
outcomes have been rare and shouldn't be
counted on as a plotting device.

It would not be credible to use melatonin in a murder or overdose scene.

What *would* be realistic? Consider these scenarios: an adult *attempted* overdose or a child's *accidental* overdose—neither with a fatal ending. These are believable plots. The number of melatonin overdoses reported during the COVID-19 pandemic, particularly in children, escalated dramatically. Why? Stress from the pandemic seemed to increase insomnia along with purchases of melatonin. This led to a large supply of the pills around homes for depressed adults to use or children to accidentally find. To keep the scene believable, though, your teen or adult character should suffer only mild symptoms, such as vomiting, nausea, headache, mild jitteriness, and mild sleepiness. Your younger character could realistically mistake the melatonin gummies for candy and eat too many. He'll have a nasty stomach ache but otherwise be fine. Or write a page-turner, with the child sedated enough that he needs medical help before he chokes on his own vomit from eating all those gummies.

Slang Terms

(Since terminology and slang terms change over time, further research is highly encouraged.)

Street names

Barbiturates: Barbs, downers
- For amobarbital: blue velvet/heaven
- For pentobarbital: yellow jackets
- For phenobarbital: goof balls
- For secobarbital: reds, pink ladies.

Benzodiazepines: Benzos, downers, tranqs (for tranquilizers)
- For alprazolam: bars, blues, chill pills, planks, xans, xanies, z-bars, zanbars
- For Valium: V's

How is it used?

Chloral hydrate was most often a liquid but sometimes in capsules. Bromides were given as a liquid. The way barbiturates and benzodiazepines are given has changed over the decades, so research the form available in the time period of your story for accuracy. Currently, medical barbiturates and benzodiazepines are given as injections, pills, or liquids. Some benzodiazepines are also used as nasal sprays. Z-drugs are typically given as pills. When benzos, barbiturates, or z-drugs are abused, pills are usually swallowed but not often snorted. Chewed benzodiazepine pills are very bitter.

If your addict tries to get a bigger high by crushing his benzos to inject, the fragments won't dissolve well in water. Injecting those fragments into his vein will cause pain and, if enough particles are injected, damage to his organs, such as his lungs and heart. Some addicts dissolve the pills in alcohol to get those particles to dissolve, but this causes severe burning during the injection, vein damage, and the risk of alcohol toxicity. Benzos are also taken together with heroin to get a combined effect, but this can be rapidly lethal. Melatonin is available in many forms: tablets, chew tablets, capsules, liquids, and gummy candies.

Now you try it

> **Writing Prompt #1** Develop an historical fiction scene for one of your own characters who's being treated for a morphine addiction and is just waking up after a weeklong bromide sleep. How does the character feel? What happens on that first day awake?

How will my character act or feel?

In general, sedatives cause feelings of relaxation and reduced anxiety, similar to alcohol. Even at recommended doses, your character will be slightly drowsy, not able to think clearly, and may be giddy. At higher doses, she can be blissfully high, dizzy, clumsy, and unsteady. Many of these drugs can create a tired hangover effect for several hours.

Barbiturates. Along with the typical sedative effects, barbiturates have their own deadly risks. High doses will cause your character to pass out and her breathing to slow to a stop. She'll die from a lack of oxygen if you don't get her emergency medical help. But since there are no antidotes for a barbiturate overdose, the only treatment possible will be to help support her breathing and other life functions until the drugs wear off. She might even need to be on a ventilator. If she survives but was without oxygen long enough, your character may suffer brain damage with permanent disabilities (see the appendix).

Is your character addicted to barbiturates? Withdrawal symptoms, beginning anywhere from twelve to forty-eight hours after her last dose, can begin as restlessness, tremors, anxiety, agitation, sweating, insomnia, and disturbing, vivid dreams. This can escalate to include hallucinations or delusions. Your character can lapse into a coma, choke on vomit during a severe seizure, or die from lethal drops in her breathing rate and blood pressure.

Benzodiazepines. In addition to sedative effects, benzos will cause your character to have amnesia or pockets of memory loss about the events that occur between the time the drug is taken until it wears off. If you're looking for a light-hearted scene, amnesia offers some options. Your protagonist may repeat the same story (several times) on her way home from a medical procedure after being sedated with a benzodiazepine. Or a teen character high on benzos might repeat a story several times in the same afternoon, raising her mom's suspicions. The amnesia also offers more sinister options. What if a vengeful son secretly hides crushed xanies in his elderly dad's food? They'll be bitter, but your creative antagonist can figure that part out! After his dad becomes progressively confused, forgetful, and even falls a time or two, does the family decide to place him in a care home?

Keep in mind, though, the amnesia from benzodiazepines does not remove *previous* memories. For example, it's not realistic for your character's childhood to be forgotten after taking benzodiazepines. Only the events for the few hours after taking a dose will be fuzzy or completely forgotten.

Don't have your character's childhood memories wiped out from benzodiazepine amnesia.

High doses of benzodiazepines can leave a character very sedated, slurring words, staggering, and even unconscious. And you could be writing a lethal ending if she's kicking back cocktails with all those benzos. After her initial happy high, she can pass out, slip into a coma, and then stop breathing. There's an antidote, flumazenil, that can reverse a benzodiazepine overdose (see "A Word about Antidotes" in chapter 3). But if she's addicted, instead of flumazenil helping, it can send the character into rapid withdrawal, including severe, unending seizures to the point where she can't breathe. The catch here is that the fastest treatment for those seizures is ... more benzodiazepine, but the antidote will block it from working and the seizures will continue. This will be the character's last scene unless she gets emergency breathing support (such as a ventilator) until the seizures can be stopped.

Your benzodiazepine-addicted character can have dangerous seizures if the antidote, flumazenil, is used.

Withdrawal from benzodiazepines causes agitation, a fast heartbeat, trembling or shaking (tremors), anxiety, nausea, vomiting, and insomnia. It can begin within twenty-four hours, but it would be realistic for your character to not have symptoms appear for a few days or even almost a week after her last dose, depending on the benzo. So if the kids hide Granny's sleeping pills because they make her too forgetful, they'll feel horrible in a day or two when they see how miserable she feels. And it could get worse. Withdrawal from benzos can turn deadly. Granny might start hallucinating and becoming paranoid of some imaginary danger. With her blood pressure going up and her heart racing, she could have a stroke or a heart attack. But Granny could also drop to the ground from a seizure and need emergency treatment before she dies. These more dramatic symptoms happen more often during withdrawal from high doses of benzos, but they have also occurred with lower doses. And Granny *might* have been taking more pills than anyone knew.

Benzo withdrawal can be lethal for your character.

Z-drugs. Along with the benzodiazepine-like effects, your character might sleepwalk, sleep-drive (yes, accidents can happen!), or even step off of a bridge. Better yet? Your character will have no memory of these events.

Melatonin. With melatonin, your character can reasonably have absolutely no symptoms or a few mild effects, such as a mild headache, nausea, or sleepiness. Children can become sleepy even with normal doses.

As discussed, the risk of overdose with melatonin in adults is highly unlikely, but a character (especially an elderly one) could be very sensitive to the effects and become fairly sleepy for several hours. High doses in younger characters can make them *extremely* sleepy. If you're writing that *rare* scene where a child does have severe overdose symptoms, she might need to be put on a ventilator to support her breathing until the drug effects wear off.

Now you try it

> **Writing Prompt #2** As it turns out, one of the teenage grandkids visiting Granny (above) decided to take several of her sleeping pills and is beginning to get very dizzy. Develop the rest of the scene. What happens? How does the scene end?

How long will this drug affect my character?

If you're writing historical fiction, the chloral hydrate will take about thirty to sixty minutes to start working and last six to eight hours. The sleepiness and difficulty thinking with bromides can last for several days. The bromide sleep, however, will cause twenty-four-hour-a-day unconsciousness for five to seven days with your poor character slowly regaining the ability to walk normally and think clearly over the next two weeks.

Benzodiazepines often cause quick sedation (within twenty to thirty seconds after the nasal spray or injection) but can take thirty minutes for the effects to start after swallowing pills. Some benzodiazepines last about four hours, but those used as sleeping pills tend to last longer and may leave a sluggish, hangover-like feeling the next day. Z-drugs also create a strong sluggish, hangover effect.

Barbiturates can be fast acting, like thiopental injection starting within twenty to thirty seconds, or slower acting oral drugs that can take twenty minutes to begin working. Some barbiturates cause sedation for up to twelve hours, leaving your character with a sluggish, hangover effect.

Melatonin supplements take about thirty minutes to start working. No one really knows how long the pills impact sleep, however. With the minimal and inconsistent effects, your adult character should have little more than mild drowsiness.

Sample Scenario Sunny opens her dresser drawers, flipping through clothes, tossing them onto the floor. *Damn it! It has to be here.* Finally, her trembling hand lands on a baggie. As she pulls it out, her face sags. It's empty. She stares at the full bag of pills on her bed. If she sells those, Kim promised to give her all the xannies she could want. She slumps in her chair, her head in her hands, shaking. *But I need more now.* She grabs the full baggie, fingering the little blue pills. Will Kim even notice just one pill missing? Or maybe two?

Now you try it

Writing Prompt #3 Continue writing the scene with Sunny (above). What happens? Does she take some of Kim's pills? Or does she steal them all? What happens when Kim finds out?

15

STIMULANTS

Stimulants offer many plot options and surprise twists—from death by caffeine (yes, this can happen!) to methamphetamine addiction.

Because of the vast number of stimulants, this chapter focuses on a few so prominent in society that authors can invoke readers' expectations to help build scene tension—or surprise them with an unexpected ending. Here you will learn how to believably subject your character to a caffeine overdose, the risks of abusing "study buddies," the life-altering dangers of methamphetamine, and the enticing yet dangerous world of cocaine.

CAFFEINE

Brief History/Social Context

Caffeine has been one of the most accepted drugs in society for centuries, although how it's used has drastically changed over the centuries and varies by culture. For example, if your scene takes place in the 1970s in Spain, we'll see your character seated at a cafe, sipping a cup of espresso. Surprisingly, that scene is still realistic in modern Spain. Move this contemporary scene to the US, and now that character is at a drive-thru ordering an iced latte with a double espresso shot for himself *and* his son before zipping his teen off to school.

Caffeine is a natural stimulant found in coffee beans and tea leaves. Medically, it has many uses, including treating headaches, counteracting sedation from pain medications, and even helping premature babies breathe better without a ventilator. And caffeine has found its way into many common products, including alertness tablets, nonprescription diuretics, diet pills, sodas, energy drinks, and sports nutrition supplements, just to name a few.

Caffeine is so popular because it causes alertness and mental focus. But it can also cause jitteriness and insomnia. As the dose of caffeine increases,

Seizures and death can be realistic in a caffeine abuse scenario.

so does the risk of more serious effects, which can include vomiting, a rapid heartrate, high blood pressure, and seizures. In rare cases, a high dose can trigger a hidden heart condition, leading to a heart attack and death. And it's addictive.

Writing a middle-grade story? Don't be afraid to add a caffeine addiction to your protagonist's flaws. Caffeine usage in children has greatly increased—up to 70 percent of US children use caffeine as a regular part of their daily lives. But how bad can that iced latte or energy drink be for a young teenager? The American Academy of Pediatrics (AAP) recommends twelve- to eighteen-year-old teens should have no more than about one 8-ounce cup of regular coffee or two 12-ounce cans of soda per day. That's only about 100 mg of caffeine daily. But some energy drinks have as much as three times that amount of caffeine and often contain additional caffeine sources, such as guarana or green tea extracts. Even "caffeine-free" drinks can have small amounts of caffeine in them. It all adds up quickly: a morning double-shot latte, a midday can of soda, and an afternoon energy shot can add up to well over 400 mg of caffeine. So, when your teen character enters an energy drink chugging contest or takes too many caffeine pills to study for final exams, he not only risks insomnia and jitteriness but possibly triggering a heart attack. And with the amount of caffeine consumed by adults, those characters are not immune to the risks of caffeine toxicity either.

Even your middle-grade character probably has caffeine as a regular part of the day.

Caffeine use is also influenced by generational norms. Alcohol-laced coffees, such as Irish coffee, have been popular among adults as relaxing after-dinner drinks across many cultures. These are rarely meant to cause intoxication but rather to pair complimentary flavors together.

In the younger generation party scene, however, caffeinated alcoholic drinks are popular, largely due to the myth that caffeine counteracts the effects of alcohol on mental alertness and coordination. Caffeine may make the person "feel less drunk" but, in fact, mental and physical reactions will remain slowed by the alcohol with potentially deadly consequences.

It may be surprising to learn that for a brief time, caffeinated alcoholic drinks were even prepackaged and sold to US consumers. Safety concerns forced manufacturers to stop marketing them in 2010. It remains popular, however, to order espresso shots or energy drinks along with alcoholic drinks at bars and clubs. If your character is about to drive from one college graduation party to another, it's realistic for him to drink a double espresso believing it will balance out the tequila shots he drank. He'll think he's fine, but your readers will be wringing their hands, waiting for the deadly accident (see chapter 4).

Taking espresso shots while drinking alcohol can give your character a false sense of alertness, but he may be dangerously impaired.

Performance pressures in the sports world also impact the use of caffeine. For some athletes, caffeine may not only be added to many workout supplements but caffeinated tablets or powders are also frequently used. And mistakes happen. Deaths have occurred from measuring errors involving concentrated caffeine powder or liquid, where a single teaspoon can contain roughly the equivalent of twenty to thirty cups of coffee, forcing the Food and Drug Administration (FDA) to warn the public against their use.

Slang Terms

(Since terminology and slang terms change over time, further research is highly encouraged.)

Street names

Joe, java, go-go juice, morning fix, morning jolt

Weaving the Plot

How is it used?

Caffeinated drinks, including coffees, teas, energy shots, and energy drinks are currently the most popular way to take caffeine. But caffeine tablets, diet pills (often labeled "metabolism booster"), concentrated powders, and sports nutrition products such as energy gels and gummies packed with caffeine are all widely used. And caffeine isn't just abused by itself. It's sometimes taken together with prescription stimulants (like Adderall) for an energetic, buzzy high.

Even a character that's a patient in a hospital might be given caffeine. He might be given a can of caffeinated soda to offset the sedation from pain medications. Injected caffeine may be used to ward off a headache from a lumbar puncture.

There are also countless creams and lotions that contain caffeine. But since this drug doesn't cross through the skin into the body, don't have a character become jittery from slathering on caffeinated cellulite cream before going to work.

Now you try it

> **Writing Prompt #1** Develop a caffeine habit for one of your characters. Would the character be more likely to drink cheap instant coffee? Expensive cappuccinos? Or take caffeine pills? What's the driving force behind the caffeine use? (You'll use this information in Writing Prompt #2.)

How will my character act or feel?

Caffeine increases alertness. In addition, it can cause tremors, jitteriness, agitation, acid reflux, heart burn and a fast heartbeat. If your teen character just chugged a double-espresso latte before his final exam, he'll be squirming in the chair waiting for a bathroom break since caffeine increases the urge to urinate. Or did a high school athlete have a couple of energy drinks before afternoon practice? He'll be energetic and talkative at practice but might have trouble sleeping that night, leaving him irritable and tired the next day.

Did a character drink several energy drinks at a party? He can be described as very chatty, restless, anxious, agitated, shaky, nauseous, and even vomiting. Need to escalate the danger? If he was goaded into an energy drink chugging contest, caffeine intoxication is a real danger, including a racing heart, racing thoughts, and agitation. His hands should noticeably tremble when he's holding a drink. He'll be dizzy, sweaty, and confused. If he does have a heart condition or has been secretly abusing prescription stimulants, that racing heart can turn deadly. The other characters (and your readers) will be shocked when he clutches his chest, his face contorted in pain, and collapses from a heart attack. If you need him to survive to the next scene, instead of a heart attack, consider having him suffer a seizure. He'll be very shaky, anxious, and confused before collapsing, his muscles spasming and twitching. Foam may even be trickling from his mouth.

Energy drink chugging contests can set a character up for a heart attack.

Withdrawal from caffeine is uncomfortable but thankfully not deadly. Your character will suffer insomnia, irritability, exhaustion, poor concentration, and nasty headaches starting a day or two after refraining from caffeine. He'll feel lousy, like he's dragging through the day, for several days before symptoms subside. The quick remedy, of course, would be more caffeine, putting your character back into the cycle of needing it to function.

Is your character sick of the way coffee makes him feel but needs a way to stay alert? He might start considering using other stimulants, like Adderall or methylphenidate (Ritalin), to help him function (see "Prescription Stimulants" in this chapter).

Now you try it

> **Writing Prompt #2** Your character from Writing Prompt #1 is in an interview for an important new job opportunity. Write the scene, knowing the character took plenty of caffeine on the way to the interview to be sharp.

How long will this drug affect my character?

The effects of caffeine start shortly after it's taken (about ten minutes when swallowed, within a few minutes if injected). Effects can last several hours in people unused to caffeine, but those who regularly take it may barely notice the effects unless the dose is fairly high. Withdrawal effects, such as headache and insomnia, can begin within one to two days and last several days to a week.

PUTTING IT ALL TOGETHER

> **Sample Scenario #1** Kaden's stomach was gurgling, threatening to send everything up. He swallowed hard, fighting back the foul taste. He stared at the last two energy drinks waiting for him and the row of expectant faces urging him to chug. With a trembling hand, he quickly tilted the next drink into his mouth, choking down the sickening sweetness. Before he could vomit, he grabbed the final can and chugged, slamming the empty container onto the table. His triumphant smile faded as the row of faces blurred, his head swirling.
>
> **Sample Scenario #2** The bartender sets the tequila shot in front of her. "Last one," he says. "Can't sell you no more tonight."
>
> Damn! She was just getting a good buzz. And she was perfectly fine. She'd already had a triple espresso to make sure. She fumbles for her keys, swigs the shot, and weaves toward the door. Well, there are plenty of other places to party. This place is getting boring, anyway.

Now you try it

COCAINE

Brief History/Social Context

Does your character with a high-level executive job need help getting through her eighty-hour work week? A hit of cocaine may be *just* the burst of energy she needs. Cocaine is a well-known addictive stimulant. Along with that burst of energy comes a euphoria and a boost of confidence. Realistically, your character can snort cocaine periodically at social events, use it to soften the "come down" off of other drug highs, or be overcome with cravings so badly that she's willing to prostitute for her next hit (dose). Your protagonist's cocaine habit can eventually lead to depression, a heart attack, a stroke, or even death. And while cocaine used to be a status symbol associated with the rich and famous of society, the costs have dropped over the decades making it believably used by a wider array of characters.

Cocaine can give your character a burst of energy, increased confidence . . . or a stroke.

While cocaine is famously known as an illicit drug, most people don't realize it was originally used as an anesthetic. The medical benefits of cocaine have been known as far back as one thousand years ago when the Amara Indians in Peru discovered the coca plant. In the 1500s, Incans chewed coca leaves or steeped them to make tea to ward off altitude sickness. Even today, some Incan natives in Peru encourage visitors to chew these leaves when hiking at high altitudes along the Inca Trail to Machu Picchu. Coca leaves have also long been used to decrease fatigue and hunger, enhance mood, and act as a digestive aid. These leaves, however, don't cause the high associated with cocaine abuse.

It wasn't until drug companies expanded research into South America in the mid-1800s that the numbing properties of cocaine were discovered, opening the door to a new era in medicine. Within a few decades of discovery, cocaine was already being used as an anesthetic nerve block.

It wasn't long after the general public realized cocaine's impact on mood and energy that it became a popular additive in wellness tonics and energy drinks. Most well-known, perhaps, is cocaine's use to enhance the flavor of the original Coca-Cola soda. Another cocaine-containing drink, Vin Mariani, also became popular, with home recipes for this wine surfacing around 1860. Cocaine was also used to relieve tooth pain.

For a story set in the late 1800s, cocaine would have been widely accepted in society.

Your cocaine-using character during this historical time period would not be arrested or considered a dangerous drug user. At the time, cocaine was thought to be safe. Even Sigmund Freud touted its benefits and published his findings that cocaine was not addictive. Unfortunately, he was wrong, and Freud, along with several other prominent physicians, eventually suffered from cocaine addiction. As reports of abuse and toxicity increased, laws were passed in the US by the mid-1900s to restrict cocaine to certain medical uses. As a result, pharmaceutical companies began the search for less addictive anesthetics, and Coca-Cola reformulated its popular soda beverage to the current cocaine-free recipe. Nevertheless, cocaine abuse has continued. It gained momentum in the 1970s, and the discovery of crack cocaine in the 1980s further accelerated abuse. Crack offered a much cheaper way to smoke cocaine, while offering the same intense high achieved by injecting the drug. This made cocaine accessible to many people that would shy away from injecting a drug.

Authors should become familiar with the various forms of cocaine that were used during the historical setting of their story, as that will impact how it should be portrayed and what terminology should be used. For example, in a 1970s setting, a character might "freebase" cocaine, whereas a poor 1980s character would more likely smoke crack.

The choice of crack or cocaine powder for a scene will be impacted by the historical setting and a character's socioeconomic status.

Did you know that cocaine is still used in modern medicine? It can be used in emergency rooms to numb wounds for stitches. It also helps stop potentially severe bleeds during nose and mouth surgery. Cocaine-soaked gauze can be packed into a nose to stop a severe bleed. Although this is very effective, nose-packing with cocaine solutions has sometimes led to dizziness, difficulty thinking clearly, a fast heart rate, and high blood pressure.

If the risks of cocaine don't escalate your protagonist's struggle enough, the prevalence of tainted street drug supplies may add the tension you're looking for. While cocaine powder has long been "cut" (diluted) to extend the supplies, increasingly dangerous drugs are being used in this process. Drugs such as fentanyl or methamphetamine are added to increase both the high and product demand. But buyers are often unaware of these additives and the increased risk of death they create (see "Fentanyl" in chapter 13).

Cocaine cut with fentanyl can add a page-turning plot twist

For authors looking for a more in-depth history of cocaine, consider reading *A Brief History of Cocaine* by S. B. Karch and *An Anatomy of Addiction: Sigmund Freud, William Halsted, and the Miracle Drug, Cocaine* by Howard Markel.

Slang Terms

(Since terminology and slang terms change over time, further research is highly encouraged.)

Street names

- For cocaine: blow, C, Charlie, coca, coke, flake, nose blow, nose candy, snow, toot, white Christmas, yayo
- For crack cocaine: candy, rock

Other terms

- Banging: injecting cocaine (also "mainlining" or "slamming").
- Blow: powdered coke, as in "I scored some blow."
- Blowing (tooting) coke: snorting lines of cocaine up the nose, often using a straw-like device (such as a rolled-up dollar bill). The powder may also be sniffed off of a spoon, fingertip, or other small tool.
- Bump: a small amount of cocaine snorted off the tip of an instrument, like a key or a small spoon, as in "do a bump."
- Butt rocket: inserting cocaine into the rectum.
- Crack: the most addictive form of cocaine. It's the result of cocaine that's been chemically treated to create a more heat stable form. Crack chunks are broken off of the small, plastic-looking, whitish-to-light-rose-colored rock, placed into a crack pipe, and smoked. It may also be heated on a piece of foil to smoke.
- Crack head: a crack addict.

- Crack lung: lung damage with hemorrhaging that may occur within a day or two after smoking crack, even after the first use. The symptoms progress rapidly and can include cough, chest pain, severe shortness of breath, difficulty breathing, gasping for air (air hunger), blue-tinged lips and fingernails, and death.
- 8-ball of coke: ⅛-ounce of coke, as in "I scored an 8-ball."
- Fiending: the agitated, desperate state of wanting more coke to keep from losing the current high; can result in users looking for any bits of coke that might be left on wrappers, tables, or even dropped on the floor to smoke or rub onto their gums. A nasal flush with water might be used to force any remaining snorted coke further into the sinuses.
- Hitting the slopes: doing coke.
- Lines of coke: long, thin mounds of coke powder placed parallel on a flat surface. These are snorted through a tube, such as a straw or rolled dollar bill, as in "I did a couple of lines."
- Mainlining: injecting cocaine into veins.
- Rails: lines of cocaine, as in "do a rail" or "ride the rails."
- Skiing: snorting coke.
- Smoke a bowl: inhaling cocaine.
- Speedball: usually a combination of a stimulant (like cocaine) and heroin or other opiate, either injected simultaneously or in sequence; benzodiazepines or barbiturates may also be combined with the cocaine in a speedball.
- The drips: the continuous drip of bitter or foul-tasting mucous down the throat after snorting cocaine; some users admit to liking the taste since they associate it with a high, as in "I was railin' last night and got the drips so bad."

Weaving the Plot

How is it used?

Lines of cocaine powder are snorted rapidly off of a surface through a straw-like device, such as a rolled-up dollar bill, placed at the nose while moving quickly along the line. Or the character may just decide to pinch off one side of her nose and snort up the line, although this is less efficient and can leave powder reside on her nose. She may snort "bumps" off of her fingertip or a small spoon. She won't want to waste a drop, so any remaining powder on the tray (or elsewhere) will be rubbed onto her gums. The bitter tasting powder will leave her tongue, gums, and throat slightly numb (cocaine is, after all, an anesthetic).

If the coke powder is moist ("wet"), a knowledgeable character may decide to "hot plate" it first, warming it on a hot surface to dry the powder out enough to snort. This drying process may magnify the chemical odor of the coke, leaving it smelling like gasoline or paint thinner. Once dry, the character can take any readily available tool, such as a knife or a credit card, to break up any clumps and shape lines to snort.

Coke powder can also be injected after being diluted in water. Freebase cocaine, however, is smoked by using a pipe (often glass), then heated to create a vapor to inhale. In some countries, a cocaine paste is smoked.

Crack is chemically treated cocaine that forms a whitish-to-clear solid rock crystal that's smoked. Small chunks are broken off and heated, often in a crack pipe, to create vapors to inhale. The heated crystal makes a crackling sound, giving it the nickname "crack," and leaves a burnt plastic smell in the air.

Add a burnt plastic smell to a scene that involves smoking crack.

Cocaine is often used together with other drugs to balance the overall effects, such as to offset the drowsiness from alcohol or marijuana. For example, at a binge-drinking college party, characters could realistically snort periodic lines of cocaine to stay awake and party longer. It's equally realistic to have a scene where cocaine is snorted to help revive the energy of a fading party. Opioids or sedatives might be taken to dampen the agitation caused by cocaine. And if your character is "speedballing," she'll either blend the cocktail of different drugs in the same syringe to inject simultaneously or inject them one right after the other. The outcome of speedballing is unpredictable and puts your character at risk of overdose or death. Sadly, numerous famous actors and musicians have died from speedballing. Some have survived with long-term impairments from a stroke or heart attack. Since coke can enhance sexual desire but impair erections, it's sometimes used with drugs that treat erectile dysfunction, such as sildenafil (Viagra). This can greatly increase the risk of a stroke or a heart attack, however.

Now you try it

> **Writing Prompt #1** Develop a scene revealing the unexpected cocaine habit of one of your own characters. Decide the setting: is the character at a club? A private party? Or maybe using it at home? Would this character be more likely to smoke crack? Snort coke? Inject it? (You'll continue this scene in Writing Prompt #2.)

How will my character act or feel?

After rubbing cocaine on her gums or lips, a bitter taste will coat your character's mouth, and those areas will rapidly become tingly and numb. If she does this regularly, her gums will develop ulcers. With snorting coke, the character's nose will burn slightly and drip, causing her to repeatedly sniff and wipe her hand across her nose. If she injects cocaine or smokes crack, her intense rush, often described as similar to a sexual orgasm, will start within seconds. The rush will fill her head with a loud ringing or rhythmic thudding sound. If she decides to snort instead, she'll have a high without that intense rush.

No matter how the character takes a hit of cocaine, the high will be pleasurable. Her body will be numb, her mouth dry, and her heart pounding. Cocaine will make her feel restless, amazingly alert, self-confident, and more chatty or sociable than usual. The feeling has been described as a burst of superhuman energy and confidence. She may become arrogant and overly bold, leading to poor, sometimes risky, decisions. Other behavior changes can include angry outbursts, agitation, and paranoia. Cocaine can also increase her sex drive. When the cocaine wears off, the crash can leave her feeling very sluggish, depressed, withdrawn, and less confident, making her believe she needs more cocaine.

Does your character want to keep her high going? She can binge on her coke until her supply is exhausted. She may be snorting coke every ten minutes, even though she's still high from the last hit. During the binge, the cocaine can cause an accelerated heart rate and profuse sweating. And with no appetite, she won't bother to eat. After repeatedly using coke throughout the evening, she'll finally become "cracked out." At this stage, she'll be utterly miserable, unable to get another good high. Her nose will be extremely stuffy and possibly even drip blood from the irritated tissue. She'll be "fiending," wanting more blow so badly that she resorts to desperate actions to get another hit. In her darkest moment, your character can find herself crawling on the floor, desperately looking for any dropped bits of coke to snort and realize how far she's fallen. Her revelation will be reinforced as she faces even more misery during her inevitable post-binge crash, including agitation, headache, body ache, stomach discomfort, insomnia, depression, and massive physical exhaustion. She still might make bad choices, though, and take some sedatives or smoke a blunt (marijuana cigarette) to soften the crash.

The crash after a cocaine binge can spin your character into depression.

Users often admit they're constantly trying to achieve the intense feeling of their first cocaine high, but it never happens again. It becomes a lie they chase by continuing to use coke. Over time, larger and larger doses are needed to get high, eventually causing an overdose risk. Even with the cost of cocaine decreasing recently, the constant need for another hit can become very expensive. Your character may turn to prostitution, stealing, selling drugs, or going into debt to buy more. With little money left for food, she can plausibly develop malnutrition and long-term nutrition-related health issues, like a permanent movement disorder. This can also lend itself to a character trait that's part of her backstory.

Your character faces many other risks by using cocaine. If she's been regularly using cocaine, she can develop paranoid behavior, even when not high, such as peering out windows to see if she's being followed. Does she live in a hot climate? Cocaine-induced high blood pressure can stop her body from naturally cooling down, causing a rapid rise in body temperature in hot weather. So, when your character's car runs out of gas along a desert road, the walk in the arid heat to find a gas station while still high on cocaine could cause heat stroke and death.

Needle-sharing puts your protagonist at risk of contracting blood-carried diseases, such as hepatitis or HIV (Human Immunodeficiency Virus). Needle "track marks" on her forearms, can become red, sore, and infected.

Regularly snorting coke causes nosebleeds and a loss of smell. Eventually, snorting creates a permanent hole in the cartilage between the nostrils. In addition, as the cocaine-tainted mucous drips down the back of your character's throat, it can create ulcers that make swallowing painful.

Smoking crack will create small crusty burns on the character's fingers or lips from the pipe. It can also cause "crack lung," a life-threatening condition that can occur within forty-eight hours even with the first high. Crack lung evolves rapidly, causing fever, cough, lung damage, severe shortness of breath, and the hemorrhaging of blood into the lungs. If your character gets crack lung, she'll die without emergency treatment. And for an asthmatic character, smoking crack can trigger a severe attack.

Crack lung can be rapidly deadly for your character.

Cocaine has long-term effects in chronic users that can include memory loss, poor concentration, depression, aggressive behavior, tremors, paranoia, loss of smell (especially from snorting), or abnormal heart rhythms. It can also leave your character's heart muscle so damaged that a hit of cocaine can trigger a heart attack.

You would think with all the effects of cocaine, that your character would go into withdrawal if she can't get more hits. However, cocaine doesn't cause typical physical withdrawal symptoms, such as shaking, vomiting, or body cramps. But your character can become agitated, mentally sluggish, lose her sense of pleasure from life, and feel depressed.

With huge variations in drug purity, overdoses can unexpectedly occur due to a more potent supply. Overdose symptoms can include severe agitation, hallucinations, paranoia, seizures, and possibly a stroke or heart attack. And for one final twist option, like so many other street drugs, cocaine is increasingly laced with potentially fatal amounts of fentanyl. The fentanyl can be your coke-snorting character's unexpected demise, as her breathing rapidly comes to a painful stop (see "Fentanyl" in chapter 13).

Now you try it

> **Writing Prompt #2** Continue the scene from Writing Prompt #1. Describe how your character behaves and feels while high on coke. Can you end the scene with a page-turner?

How long will this drug affect my character?

Unlike the instant high seen on some shows, the high from snorting cocaine starts slowly over several minutes and can last about thirty minutes. Smoking crack or injecting cocaine, however, causes a rapid high (rush) within seconds but lasting as short as five to ten minutes. No matter how your character takes it, the increase in her alertness, confidence, and heart rate can last several more hours after the initial rush has disappeared.

PUTTING IT ALL TOGETHER

> **Sample Scenario** I stare at the line of empty red Solo cups on the counter, my head resting on my hand. I'll puke if I drink any more. My eyes are heavy and begin to flutter closed. Mike fumbles with something behind me, then cusses. The keg must be empty. I hear a thump next to me. Carmen has tossed a baggie of white powder on the counter.
>
> "Time to get this party started," she laughs.

Now you try it

METHAMPHETAMINE

Brief History/Social Context

Interested in weaving methamphetamine into your story? Be prepared to develop either a very dark character or a heart-wrenching redemption arc. Either way, lives will be destroyed. Methamphetamine ("meth") causes a rapid, explosive euphoria, triggering brain chemicals that create intense drug cravings. Meth is one of *the* most addictive drugs, contributing significantly to violent crime in America. Disturbingly, almost 80 percent of crime in one California county has been estimated to be methamphetamine related. Why? Because the drug cravings can be so strong that addicts will do anything for their next hit (dose), including prostitution, assault, robbery, child abuse and endangerment (think trafficking), and murder. Meth can also cause violent behavior, hallucinations, and psychotic events. Ultimately, users can die from a stroke or heart attack. Neighborhoods suffer collateral damage from local meth production, with gun violence, the risk of home lab explosions, and even waterway contamination by the toxic waste byproducts from cooking meth.

Your meth-addicted character might do anything for another hit of meth, from stealing to murder.

Like many abused drugs, methamphetamine started out as a valid medical treatment. Beginning in the early 1900s, it was used for alertness, as a nasal decongestant, and for weight loss. By the mid-1900s, abuse of methamphetamine had grown significantly and continues today. Drug traffickers responded to this new potential market by developing a rapid method to make large supplies of an even more intense "boosted meth." Using simple household cleaners and common nonprescription decongestants, like pseudoephedrine, clandestine labs used this "shake and bake" method to create what became known as crystal meth. In response, to curb access to pseudoephedrine, ephedrine, and other potential ingredients, states restricted access to these drugs. As of 2006, these decongestants must be stored behind a pharmacist's counter or in a locked cabinet and can only be purchased with photo identification, with a strict thirty-day purchase limit. As an additional barrier, manufacturers repackaged pseudoephedrine into blister pill packs, instead of bulk bottles. Authors can research the Methamphetamine Act of 1996 and the Combat Methamphetamine Epidemic Act of 2005 for more details. As the battle to make meth continued, illicit labs responded to the new laws by sending workers to multiple stores to collect pills (a process called "smurfing"), then pooling the purchases to make meth. To counter that, some states further restricted pseudoephedrine access by requiring a prescription for its purchase. Undeterred however, clandestine labs continue to find alternate chemicals to use in meth production.

Many meth users are more interested in getting the next high than which production method was used. However, some users are very well versed in the differences in potency and the high achieved from various chemical production processes. To create authentic dialogue for characters discussing this, writers are encouraged to research online chat forums, where countless threads offer realistic views into the terms, language, and culture associated with the impact of different ingredients.

If your character is a meth cook, his access to raw chemicals will differ depending on the historical setting of the story. One set in 2020 should not involve him buying bulk bottles of pseudoephedrine, but in 1990 it could. In 2010, it's realistic to have a crew of "smurfs" collecting pseudoephedrine at stores, littering parking lots with emptied blister pill packs, and returning filled collection bottles to your cook, in hopes for a hit of meth as payment. Or maybe your character is just a small-time cook, making his own supply in his tool shed to share with friends. With the complexity of the production process, it would not be recommended to get too deep into the details in a scene, unless you are very well-versed in the language.

Your character could be a "smurf" or a small-time meth cook.

Would you be surprised to know methamphetamine is approved to treat pediatric attention-deficit-hyperactivity-disorder (ADHD) and severe obesity? While still available to prescribe, other medications are more often used. For example, it's rarely prescribed for ADHD anymore, due to the availability of other drugs that are considered safer. Unfortunately, many of these other drugs are also amphetamines, such as Ritalin or Adderall, and are

Prescription stimulant abuse could be a road to meth addiction for your character.

abused (see "Prescription Stimulants" in this chapter). So, while it's not likely your character will be prescribed meth for ADHD, he *could* get prescribed a different amphetamine. This may be perfectly fine, unless he begins to abuse his medication. Abuse of prescription stimulants has become a bridge to meth addiction for some. *Now* you've fueled your character's conflicts.

Currently, methamphetamine is made in countless small, illicit labs across the US. These clandestine mini-kitchens, using the "shake and bake" or other production variations, are hidden in motels, apartments, and even private homes. Meth is also brought into the US across the southern border from Mexican "superlabs" by smugglers that have developed creative ways to sneak past border scrutiny. For example, meth has been found hidden stuffed in holes drilled into stacks of tortillas. Individual people ("mules") are also recruited to smuggle meth (and other drugs) into the US. If one of your characters is a mule, he's likely been forced to swallow dozens of meth-filled packets, risking his life, if even just one bursts (see chapter 8).

Meth may also be cut (diluted) with talcum powder or sugar to extend the supplies and increase profits. Unfortunately for your character, these additives can clump in his veins when he injects the meth, causing skin ulcers or blocking blood flow to his heart or brain, ending in death. Supplies are also being cut with other drugs, such as cocaine, heroin, or fentanyl. This not only extends the batches but adds a "boost" to the high, increasing product demand. Traffickers don't focus on careful mixing, though, causing some batches to contain potentially lethal amounts of the "boost." Accidental fentanyl overdoses from tainted street drugs have drastically increased over the last few years. This unfortunate reality can help you craft a surprise twist, when the character your readers have been rooting for relapses into drug use, takes a hit of meth, and dies from a fentanyl overdose (see "Fentanyl" in chapter 13).

Overall, meth has become much less expensive over the decades, fueling its increased use. In fact, the prices have dropped so much that meth is even added to *other* street drugs, such as counterfeit Adderall pills (see "Prescription Stimulants" in this chapter). Despite the drop in cost, your meth-addicted character can lose everything—his family, his job, his home—in his desperation to get his next fix of meth.

Slang Terms

(Since terminology and slang terms change over time, further research is highly encouraged.)

Street names

crank, fire, glass, go fast, ice (crystal meth), shards, speed (usually a powder form of amphetamine), Tina (crystal meth)

Other terms

- Base: a thick yellowish-brown oily form of meth injected or swallowed; also "wax" or "paste."
- Blowing clouds: smoking meth, as in "I was at Trey's last night blowin' clouds."
- Booty bump: rectal use of a drug (also "butt rocket," "boofed," or "plugging"), as in "I never slam meth, just booty bump it."
- Bump: a small amount of meth, usually snorted, as in "I bump meth before work every morning."
- Crack back: remaining meth in a pipe that was melted, which when cooled down creates a snowflake-like solid.
- 8-Ball: ⅛ of an ounce of drug.
- Ice: historically a purer form of meth, usually smoked or injected (also "glass," "shards"). Complaints of low purity and a less satisfactory high have increased with recipe changes over the years.
- Puddle: the liquified portion of meth in a pipe bowl.
- Rolling (rocking) the bowl: a pipe bowl is rolled over a flame to avoid burning the meth and generate a vapor to inhale, as in "I was rollin' a bowl last night."
- Speedballing: general term for getting high by simultaneously taking an opioid and a stimulant, such as combining meth and heroin.

Weaving the Plot

How is it used?

Meth is snorted, smoked, injected into a vein (slammed, mainlined), booty bumped (inserted into the rectum), or swallowed. Before injecting, powdered meth is dissolved, sometimes in the baggie it was purchased in. The liquid should be heated to avoid infection, but this isn't always done. The diluted meth is then pulled into a syringe, usually through a cotton ball or other filter to help remove fragments. Smoking meth is popular because it avoids injections but still gives a rapid high. When smoking crystal meth, the drug will resemble small, translucent glass fragments (shards) or bluish-white rocks. Your character will generally place his meth into a glass pipe and heat it over a flame. Slowly rolling the pipe bowl will keep the meth from burning, allowing the liquified meth "puddle" to flow to the cooler side of the bowl and releasing the vapor for him to slowly inhale. Once the flame is removed, the meth resolidifies ("cracks back"). Instead of a pipe, meth is sometimes simply burned on a piece of aluminum foil and inhaled using a straw or cupped hands to guide the vapor toward the nose. Powder meth (speed) can be snorted or diluted to use for booty bumps.

Your character may take meth bumps before work in the morning, low-dose hits throughout an evening at a party, or go on a meth binge lasting several days. With binges, he'll keep taking more meth hits to avoid the come down (losing the high).

Now you try it

> **Writing Prompt #1** Develop the backstory for one of your own characters with a history of meth addiction. What drove the character to use meth the first time? Was it prescription stimulant abuse or a friend's bad influence? Is addiction still a problem? Or is the character now a recovered addict, hoping to help others avoid the same fate? (You'll use this information in Writing Prompt #2.)

How will my character act or feel?

Smoking or injecting meth will immediately give your character an intense, exhilarating, high, making him feel like he's floating, his body tingling everywhere. The rush has been compared to an overwhelming orgasmic sensation. He'll be suddenly alert, hyperactive, talkative, and socially confident. While using meth he won't sleep or have an appetite, since meth suppresses hunger. He may find himself hyperfocused on a single task, like cleaning the bathroom for hours. Meth can make him act superior and aggressively assertive toward others. And it can cause him to be very sexually aroused, sometimes to the point of engaging in sex for hours. Depending on the dose, he can be nauseous, vomit, have severe tremors (shakes), be drenched in sweat, tightly clench his jaws, and grind his teeth, potentially cracking them.

It's realistic to have your character go from trying meth to wanting it to *needing* it. As your character begins to use more meth and becomes addicted, his personality will begin to change—subtly at first, then drastically. The initial energetic high and social confidence from a periodic hit (or two) can turn into a regular habit. As tolerance grows (where more meth is needed to get the same high) so will the cost of his habit.

Your character's room and clothes may have a sweet odor, similar to burnt marshmallows, burnt plastic, or sweet almond oil, from smoking meth. Some users suggest the smell varies and may be almost absent, depending on drug purity and what chemicals were used to cut the batch.

Meth can quickly take your character from trying it to wanting it to *needing* it.

If your character goes on a meth binge, he'll constantly be on the go and not able to sit and relax. But he'll get progressively exhausted and stuck in a repeating cycle of meth high, meth stimulation, no sleep, and agitation, followed by more meth. At this point, he may be "tweaking" (sometimes "tweaking out"). Tweaking is the point when someone has been overstimulated so long by meth that they're no longer able to control their public actions and are openly displaying exaggerated behaviors of a meth high. You can portray your character with extreme excitability, incessant loud talking, a rocking back and forth motion, and even small, repetitive, jerking body movements. His skin may be covered in open, bleeding wounds from continually scratching at bugs he thinks are crawling on him. In addition, because of the overstimulation, any meth that he does take won't give him the high he craves, leaving him highly agitated and becoming openly aggressive. These exhaustive stretches without sleep can trigger hallucinations and aggressive paranoia. Your character may believe he's being followed or watched, making him act dangerously and irrationally (such as bringing out a gun for protection), creating the opportunity for a great tension-building scene.

Eventually, your character will run out of meth (and the money for more) and crash. He'll be overcome with severe emotional and physical exhaustion, lash out in anger at others, and become depressed. He may sleep for days, but it will be poor sleep, filled with disturbing dreams, including visions driven by meth cravings. He'll wake feeling so horrible that he'll vow never to touch meth again, only to be lured into the lie of another hit. It may not be today or tomorrow. But it's realistic to have your character pulling his life back together, only to be tempted with meth by his new girlfriend. And this is where you get to choose how the character tackles his inner demon. Does he fall into the grips of meth again? Or is he strong enough to walk away from the meth . . . and her.

Depression can be triggered when your character crashes after a meth binge.

If a character is cooking meth, his neighbors may become suspicious of the pervasive odor similar to window cleaner, ammonia, or cat urine around his home from the chemicals. Other telltale signs of a home meth kitchen can include dark curtain-draped windows, water hoses leading into the house, and a constant cycle of visitors throughout the day and night.

Meth users rapidly begin to look much older and gaunt. Authors can research online photos that compare the images of people before and after the ravages of meth to see how to accurately portray these drastic changes. Use the keywords *meth age progression* and *meth mouth*. It's not an exaggeration for a character's handsome senior yearbook photo to morph into an almost unrecognizable police mugshot with scabs, oozing wounds, "meth mouth" (broken and missing teeth in rotting gums), sunken cheeks, and dark circles under vacant eyes.

Chronic meth use can eventually cause your character to have hallucinations, paranoid delusions, and violent behavior even when he isn't high. He can suffer memory impairment, which can be permanent. And poor circulation will cause his fingers and toes to be painfully cold. Infected sores can develop at his injection sites or he can contract serious diseases from sharing needles with other addicts, such as hepatitis or HIV. A stroke or heart attack is also a sad but realistic end to your meth-addicted character.

Your character can suffer "meth mouth," sore-covered skin, and paranoid delusions.

Is it believable to have a chronic meth-using character hide his habit from others? Well, *maybe*. Self-described "functional" meth users say they're able to shield their families and friends from their meth use by working hard to avoid the associated physical changes. If this is your character, he'll fight off the impulse to take meth in the afternoon or evening to avoid insomnia and be vigilant about eating to avoid losing weight. He'll take lower doses of meth when he's around other people and carefully monitor his behavior. And he'll regularly visit the dentist. "Functional" meth users say they have known people that have convincingly hidden their habit for years. Other users say that's impossible.

How realistic is it to have your character addicted after a single meth hit (dose)? Actually, *very* realistic. Highly potent meth causes the release of excessive amounts of a pleasure chemical in the brain called dopamine, leaving even some first-time users emotionally empty and craving more. Less potent meth causes a slower dopamine release, lengthening the process of developing addiction. but there's no specific number of doses that will cause meth addiction, since each person's body responds to those dopamine surges differently. So while some users swear they took many doses of meth before becoming addicted, other lament that their first dose ruined their lives as they fell headlong out of control, losing everything.

Planning to have your addicted character run out of meth? Withdrawal will make him suffer intense drug cravings, along with severe depression, anxiety, aggressive paranoia, and he'll potentially become a physical danger to others.

If addiction and recovery is your character's backstory, keep in mind that meth is one of the most difficult drugs to stop using. There are no drugs available to support withdrawal and recovery, unlike with opioid addiction. It's reasonable to have your character dramatically fighting his inner desire for meth for years (or even for life), especially in situations that remind him of past use or when he's under severe stress. No matter *how* horrible his life became while addicted, the deep cravings can haunt him. While this is the sad reality of meth addiction, it also allows for a writer to create a compelling character with strong motivation for his actions.

Recovery from meth addiction can create a moving backstory.

In a meth overdose scene, your character can suffer a racing heartbeat, nausea, vomiting, shaking, dizziness, and severe confusion. Worse symptoms can include delirium, paranoia, crazed behavior, and a body temperature high enough to damage his brain, heart, or other organs. He may collapse from a seizure, with foam dripping from his mouth as his body convulses. And your character can end up in a coma. In his final moments, he may die from a stroke, a heart attack, or organ failure.

Now you try it

> **Writing Prompt #2** With the background developed in Writing Prompt #1, write a scene of your character's typical day. How has the meth addiction shaped daily life? Do others in your character's life know about the addiction?

How long will this drug affect my character?

The intense rush of pleasure and racing heartbeat from smoking or injecting meth is almost immediate. Snorting or swallowing meth causes a less drastic, slower high within several minutes (snorting about five minutes, swallowing about twenty minutes). Initial effects from any of these methods will fade over another thirty minutes. But even after the rush is gone, many other effects can remain for twelve to twenty-four hours, such as the high energy levels, insomnia, agitation, or aggressive behavior.

The come down from a meth dose can occur over a few hours and will be milder from snorting, than from smoking or injecting it. The crash after many doses or a meth binge can last several days or longer.

PUTTING IT ALL TOGETHER

Sample Scenario #1 Ken walks out of the gas station, heading to his car, a bag of beer and chips tucked under his arm. A gaunt, dirty teenager looks up, his eyes hallowed, his skin covered in oozing sores.

"Change?" the boy pleads, reaching out a trembling hand. His weak smile exposes a row of broken, yellowed teeth.

Ken drops his bag. "Charlie?" he whispers. *It can't be. Is this Mike's son? The high school quarterback that used to live down the street?* "Charlie Carter? Is that you?"

Sample Scenario #2 "We told him not to do it. The meth, I mean," the teen told the police. "He got all shaky . . . started yelling and stuff. He even took a swing at me. That's when I knocked him out. He's been laying there ever since. He started jerking his legs around just before you showed up."

Now you try it

Writing Prompt #3 Continue the scene with Ken and Charlie, from Sample Scenario #1. How does it end? Is Ken able to take Charlie back to his parents for rehabilitation? Or does Charlie attack Ken with a hidden knife, stealing his wallet?

PRESCRIPTION STIMULANTS

(Methylphenidate [Ritalin], Amphetamine/
dextroamphetamine blend [Adderall], and More)

Brief History/Social Context

Need an energy booster that's more dangerous than caffeine pills for your characters? Many people don't realize that several drugs prescribed for

ADHD (attention deficit hyperactivity disorder) are not only amphetamines but chemical cousins to methamphetamine. These include methylphenidate (Ritalin), a combination amphetamine (Adderall), and several other brands (Vyvanse, Concerta) (see "A Note of Caution: Using Brand Names" in chapter 1).

With a long history of use in ADHD (dating back to the 1930s), these drugs have become widely accepted as safe. Unfortunately, they are also highly addictive and abused for their ability to cause a methamphetamine- or cocaine-like high with a burst of energy and self-confidence. Students and young professionals may use them to combat mental sluggishness from hangovers, to boost energy for project deadlines, or to stay awake all night to study. In fact, these pills have been dubbed "study buddies" due to the common myth that they help improve grades. And although some recreational users have found success with their "study buddies," for many, the outcome is detrimental. These drugs are also abused to help with weight loss, since they decrease appetite.

> Characters can be driven to abuse "study buddies" believing they will help improve grades.

Prescription stimulant abuse can be a realistic flaw for a wide range of character ages, from a young teen through a middle-aged adult. So, your high school student selling "Addys" (Adderall) to an eighth-grader during lunch is a believable scene. Or you can choose a fifty-year-old character who's been abusing them for years and now *needs* them to just get through the day. Abuse in older adults, however, is not as common.

It's not uncommon for people prescribed stimulants to boost (take extra dose) on days they particularly need to focus, such as during final exams. Some users say boosts help them get through the day better. But there are plenty that lament starting down the pathway of extra doses, claiming it eventually got out of control and ruined their lives. They're more likely to describe relying on the pills for long stretches of time, believing grades or work performance would improve with the extra effort and alertness. In reality, according to users, continuing to take these extra doses will result in decreased performance. With these pills, instead of finishing a term paper your character can find herself hyperfocused on one specific task, such as scrolling social media for hours. Or she might rewrite the opening paragraph of that paper over and over and over again. But the rest of the paper won't get the same attention to detail, resulting in a lousy grade. Your character can believably respond by deciding to study harder . . . which will require more pills. Eventually, when she tries to stop using the pills, her foggy brain and

Abusing prescription stimulants can lead to experimenting with cocaine or meth.

sluggish body will be the first signs of drug dependence. If she recognizes these warning signs and stops using the pills, after an initial struggle against exhaustion, life can return to normal. But taking more pills will seem like the easiest and fastest way to get control of life. Unfortunately, tolerance will occur, meaning continuously higher doses will be needed to get the same effects. This can spiral the character into a pattern of higher doses, poor sleep, poor nutrition, and decreased performance, all while heading toward addiction.

Where will your character keep getting the pills? They'll be easy to buy at school, steal from a friend, buy on social media apps, or get by prescription after faking ADHD-like symptoms. When the stimulants don't do the trick anymore, your character may be tempted to try something stronger, like cocaine or methamphetamine.

Snorting extended-release amphetamines can give your character a meth-like high . . . or kill her.

Stopping the pills once addicted will cause your character to feel horrible. She'll battle brain fog, a loss of motivation, anxiety, anger, and weight gain as her appetite returns.

The cocaine or meth-like high from these stimulants has made them some of the most popular prescription pills stolen to either abuse or sell. Snorting crushed regular pills causes a rapid energy burst and a feeling of invincibility. And snorting the crushed contents of an extended-release pill sends twelve hours of amphetamine to the brain within minutes, causing an even more intense high. This can cause an overdose with hallucinations, seizures, and sudden death. Despite this, abusers risk these dangers for the high.

Drug shortages can leave your character in unexpected withdrawal or in danger of buying fentanyl-laced counterfeit pills.

In 2022, a shortage of prescription amphetamines left many suddenly without their ADHD medication for days to weeks. Those that were prescribed stimulants for ADHD, as well as those regularly abusing them, reported a loss of daily functioning, brain fog, and an inability to focus. How could this impact your characters? A student's grades could suffer. An amphetamine abuser may hoard her supply, possibly taking half the usual dose to get by. She could try borrowing or buying some from friends, but they may be hoarding their supply, too. So, she may turn to street supplies. But buying pills from strangers carries dangerous risks. Some street supplies of prescription stimulants have been tainted with dangerous drugs such as methamphetamine. Others have contained potentially lethal amounts of fentanyl. Your character, who buys "Addys" from a link on a social media app or a stranger at a club may not realize the pills are counterfeit until it's too late. *Now* you may be writing an accidental fentanyl overdose scene (see "Fentanyl" in chapter 13).

Slang Terms

(Since terminology and slang terms change over time, further research is highly encouraged.)

Street names

Addys, diet coke, kiddie coke, poor man's coke, r-balls, smart pills, smarties, study buddy, vitamin R

Weaving the Plot

How is it used?

To treat ADHD, the short and long-acting versions of these pills may be combined to take advantage of the benefits of both. The drugs, how long they last, and the dosing schedules have changed over the decades. But one example could be an extended-release pill taken in the morning with a quick-releasing pill ("a boost") at midday. Doses taken later in the day can cause insomnia. So your character whose child forgot to take his midday dose until *after* school may be up late with an agitated, emotionally charged insomniac, wondering how she'll get through tomorrow's business presentation.

When abused, an extra pill (or two) may be taken for a quick energy burst or several pills might be taken to get high. These are swallowed or crushed to snort. They may also be plugged (inserted into the rectum). Your character can realistically use marijuana or a sedative, such as a benzodiazepine, to calm her agitation or insomnia from the stimulants.

> Some stimulant abusers take benzodiazepines or marijuana to counteract insomnia or agitation.

If she's a chronic abuser, it may be impossible for her to function in the morning before a dose. Keeping the pill bottle stored at her

Without a drug holiday, your character will need higher doses for effects; with the holiday, your character may suffer withdrawal symptoms.

bedside will allow her to take a dose as soon as she wakes up, in hopes that she'll feel better by the time she showers.

"Drug holidays" are days or weeks without doses that are used to reduce tolerance, a condition that requires increasingly higher doses to get the desired effect. ADHD treatment schedules are created to help avoid tolerance, but dose increases may still be needed over time. Without a drug holiday, chronic abusers will lose the high and sharp focus they want from taking the pills. Unless you want your character to be a sluggish, mentally exhausted mess at work or school, she should schedule her drug-free days over a weekend or during a vacation.

Now you try it

> **Writing Prompt #1** Your high school character has been under a lot of pressure to get better grades and scholarships. Develop a scene where the student finally decides to buy "study buddies" over lunch at school. (You'll use this information in Writing Prompt #2.)

How will my character act or feel?

There are many differences between all the various prescription stimulants in terms of how they make a person feel and how they're used and abused. Covering them all is beyond the scope of this book. Instead, this section will focus on the classic symptoms of these stimulants that can believably be woven into your story.

With prescription stimulants, your character will feel mentally sharp and focused with a burst of energy lasting a few hours. Swallowing longer-acting pills won't cause an energy burst, but a slower build of effects over a few hours. If your character has ADHD, these stimulants can make him function better in school and life. But no matter who's taking them, insomnia will be a problem, especially when doses are taken later in the day, and appetite suppression will lead to weight loss. And whether abused as study buddies or to help your character work long, stressful hours, she may find herself with tunnel vision, hyperfocusing on one single task for hours.

Need a plausible scenario for your character to innocently take an overdose of one of these stimulants? When she sees how much more focus she has with a *single* pill, she may be fooled into thinking that taking a few more pills will work even better. Instead, that load of stimulants will give your character a racing heart, anxiety, nausea, vomiting, and tremors (shaking). These symptoms can trigger a severe panic attack, with your character spending the night in the emergency room, sedated. A seasoned amphetamine abuser, however, would wait for the symptoms to subside instead of panicking. But if the symptoms are actually signs of a heart attack unfolding, your character may regret that choice.

A panic attack can land your character in the emergency room sedated until the amphetamines wear off.

Snorting amphetamines or taking high doses will give your character a quick, energetic high. She'll become chatty and restless, lose her appetite, and her heart will be rapidly beating. It can also cause an overwhelming anxiety attack, dizziness, and vomiting.

What can happen to your character that chronically abuses these amphetamines? She can develop aggression and hostility. Overstimulation and long periods without sleep can realistically trigger hallucinations and paranoia. She can also become dysfunctional even while taking the pills. If she stops taking the pills, once the stimulation wears off, she'll "crash," suffering severe exhaustion, anger, depression, brain fog, and poor sleep. She'll feel absolutely miserable and unable to function. This can pass over several days or become worse, with headaches, agitation, mood swings, tremors, hostility, and paranoia. Taking more pills to relieve the misery will be very tempting.

The crash after using amphetamines for a long period can be debilitating.

Does your character snort amphetamines? Include a loss of smell, continually clogged sinuses, a runny nose, nose bleeds, and even a hole between her nostrils to her list of problems.

During a drug holiday, your character will be exhausted with a foggy brain, lack of motivation, and little interest in the world. These feelings will go away over days to weeks if she stays off the pills. If she starts taking them again, eventually she'll stop getting the excited, energetic, and happy high she craves, but still need the pills to function and avoid withdrawal. She'll be stuck in a vicious cycle.

Now you try it

Writing Prompt #2 Continue the scene from Writing Prompt #1. Your character bought some Addy's from a friend, hoping to stay up all night and finish the school paper due the next day. After taking one, how does the character feel? What happens when the character begins to doze off and decides to take a couple of extra doses?

How long will this drug affect my character?

Regular tablets usually cause effects within an hour and last four to six hours. When swallowed, the extended-release pills can last eight to twelve hours. Snorting these stimulants can cause a high within minutes (five to ten), with the heightened energy and stimulation lasting as long as four to six hours. Crushed extended-release pills can cause a rapid high within five minutes, whether snorted or plugged (inserted into the rectum).

PUTTING IT ALL TOGETHER

Sample Scenario Asa rolls over, groaning, hitting the button on her alarm. Her eyes are too heavy to open, her brain foggy. *It's gonna be a rough one.* She fumbles in the dark, finding the little bottle, tipping a pill into her mouth, and swallowing. She forces herself into the shower, shoving her face into the icy cold water, waiting. *Soon. It'll kick in soon.* She waits. The energy slowly returns, her head clearing.

Now you try it

Writing Prompt #3 Write a scene where a character abusing Addys for several months takes a drug holiday for the weekend. How does the weekend unfold?

APPENDIX

POSSIBLE SYMPTOMS OF BRAIN DAMAGE FROM LOSS OF OXYGEN

Memory loss

Loss of balance

Vision loss (mild loss to total blindness)

Muscle spasms (mild twitching to severe limb spasms)

Difficulty speaking (mild to severe)

Difficulty swallowing (mild to severe,
may need to have a permanent feeding tube)

Difficulty thinking, confusion

Partial or total paralysis

NOTES

1. First Things First

Collins, Suzanne. *The Hunger Games*. New York: Scholastic, 2010.

2. Using Toxidromes to Plot That Twist

Sam Ashoo. "Toxidromes," Free Open Access Medical Education, EB Medicine, June 19, 2022, https://foamed.ebmedicine.net/rapid-reference/toxidromes/.

"Toxidromes." Florida's Poison Control Centers, accessed August 2021, https://floridapoisoncontrol.org/healthcare-professional/toxidromes.

3. A Word about Antidotes

Rzasa, Lynn R., and J. L. Galinkin. "Naloxone Dosage for Opioid Reversal: Current Evidence and Clinical Implications." *Therapeutic Advances in Drug Safety* 9, no. 1 (2017): 63–88. https://doi.org/10.1177/2042098617744161.

Sharbaf Shoar, Nazila, Karlyle G. Bistas, and Abdolreza Saadabadi. "Flumazenil." StatPearls [Internet]. Updated August 29, 2022. https://www.ncbi.nlm.nih.gov/books/NBK470180/.

Sharpless, Norman E. "Statement on Continued Efforts to Increase Availability of All Forms of Naloxone to Help Reduce Opioid Overdose Deaths." US Food and Drug Administration. September 20, 2019. https://www.fda.gov/news-events/press-announcements/statement-continued-efforts-increase-availability-all-forms-naloxone-help-reduce-opioid-overdose.

4. Alcohol

Centers for Disease Control and Prevention. "Alcohol Use." June 11, 2021. https://www.cdc.gov/nchs/fastats/alcohol.htm.

Mekonnen, Serkalem. "Rubbing Alcohol Only Looks Like Water." National Capital Poison Center. Accessed August 2021, https://www.poison.org/articles/rubbing-alcohol-only-looks-like-water.

National Institute on Alcohol Abuse and Alcoholism. "Alcohol Facts and Statistics." June 2021. https://www.niaaa.nih.gov/publications/brochures-and-fact-sheets/alcohol-facts-and-statistics.

National Institute on Drug Abuse. "Alcohol Trends & Statistics." December 15, 2020. https://www.drugabuse.gov/drug-topics/alcohol/alcohol-trends-statistics.

Peterson, Thomas, Landen Rentmeester, Bryan S. Judge, Stephen D. Cohle, and Jeffrey S. Jones. "Self-Administered Ethanol Enema Causing Accidental Death." *Case Reports in Emergency Medicine,* (November 2014): 1–3. https://doi.org/10.1155/2014/191237.

Wilson, Christopher I., Susan S. Ignacio, and Gwennaëlle A. Wilson. "An Unusual Form of Fatal Ethanol Intoxication." *Journal of Forensic Sciences* 50, no. 3 (2005): 1–3. https://doi.org/10.1520/jfs2004325.

5. Antidepressants

Bruggeman, Clare, and Carla S. O'Day. "Selective Serotonin Reuptake Inhibitor Toxicity." StatPearls, July 5, 2022. https://www.ncbi.nlm.nih.gov/books/NBK534815.

Giwa, Al, and Edwin Oey. "The Return of an Old Nemesis: Survival after Severe Tricyclic Antidepressant Toxicity, a Case Report." *Toxicology Reports,* no. 5 (2018): 357–62. https://doi.org/10.1016/j.toxrep.2018.03.009.

Hillhouse, Todd M., and Joseph H. Porter. "A Brief History of the Development of Antidepressant Drugs: From Monoamines to Glutamate." *Experimental and Clinical Psychopharmacology* 23, no. 1 (2015): 1–21. https://doi.org/10.1037/a0038550.

Khalid, Muhammad M., and Muhammad Waseem. "Tricyclic Antidepressant Toxicity." StatPearls [Internet]. July 21, 2021. https://www.ncbi.nlm.nih.gov/books/NBK430931.

King, Matthew, and Nauman Ashraf. "Tricyclic Antidepressant-Induced Anticholinergic Delirium in a Young Healthy Male Individual." *Drug Safety - Case Reports* 5, no. 1 (2018). https://doi.org/10.1007/s40800-017-0069-5.

National Institute on Drug Abuse. "Overdose Death Rates." January 29, 2021. https://www.drugabuse.gov/drug-topics/trends-statistics/overdose-death-rates.

6. Antihistamines

Borowy, Christopher S., and Pinaki Mukherji. "Antihistamine Toxicity." StatPearls [Internet]. March 12, 2021. https://www.ncbi.nlm.nih.gov/books/NBK482318.

Hedegaard, Holly, Brigham A. Bastian, James P. Trinidad, Merianne R. Spencer, and Margaret Warner. "Regional Differences in the Drugs Most Frequently Involved in Drug Overdose Deaths: United States, 2017." *National Vital Statistics Reports* 68, no. 12 (October 2019): 1–15. https://www.cdc.gov/nchs/data/nvsr/nvsr68/nvsr68_12-508.pdf.

Seger, Donna. "What is the Treatment of Antihistamine Overdose?" Tennessee Poison Center. August 26, 2020. https://www.vumc.org/poison-control/toxicology-question-week/aug-26-2020-what-treatment-antihistamine-overdose.

US Food and Drug Administration. "FDA Warns about Serious Problems with High Doses of the Allergy Medicine Diphenhydramine (Benadryl)." September 24, 2020. https://www.fda.gov/drugs/drug-safety-and-availability/fda-warns-about-serious-problems-high-doses-allergy-medicine-diphenhydramine-benadryl.

7. Bath Salts

Drug Enforcement Administration. "Bath Salts Fact Sheet." April 2020. https://www.dea.gov/sites/default/files/2020-06/Bath%20Salts-2020.pdf.

National Institute on Drug Addiction. "Bath Salts." May 3, 2021. https://teens.drugabuse.gov/drug-facts/bath-salts.

National Institute on Drug Addiction. "Synthetic Cathinones" ('Bath Salts') Drug Facts." July 6, 2020. https://www.drugabuse.gov/publications/drugfacts/synthetic-cathinones-bath-salts.

Slomski, Anita. "A Trip on 'Bath Salts' Is Cheaper Than Meth or Cocaine but Much More Dangerous. *Journal of the American Medical Association* 308 no., 23 (2012): 2445. https://doi.org/10.1001/jama.2012.34423.

TripSit Factsheets. "MDPV." Accessed May 18, 2021. https://drugs.tripsit.me/MDPV.

8. BODY PACKING

Abedzadeh, Ayoub A., Shaikh S. Iqbal, Usama Al Bastaki, and Claude Pierre-Jerome. "New Packaging Methods of Body Packers: Role of Advanced Imaging in Their Detection. A Case Study." *Radiology Case Reports* 14, no. 5 (2019): 627–33. https://doi.org/10.1016/j.radcr.2019.03.002.

Pinto, A., A. Reginelli, F. Pinto, G. Sica, M. Scaglione, F. H. Berger, L. Romano, and L. Brunese. "Radiological and Practical Aspects of Body Packing." *The British Journal of Radiology* 87, no. 1036 (2014). https://doi.org/10.1259/bjr.20130500.

Traub, Stephen J., Robert S. Hoffman, and Lewis S. Nelson. "Body Packing—the Internal Concealment of Illicit Drugs." *New England Journal of Medicine* 349, no. 26 (2003): 2519–26. https://doi.org/10.1056/nejmra022719.

Tsang, Ho K. P., Chevk K. K. Wong, and Oi F. Wong. "Radiological Features of Body Packers: An Experience from a Regional Accident and Emergency Department in Close Proximity to the Hong Kong International Airport." *Hong Kong Journal of Emergency Medicine* 25, no. 4 (2018): 202–10. https://journals.sagepub.com/doi/10.1177/1024907918770083.

United Nations Office on Drugs and Crime. "Drug Mules: Swallowed by the Illicit Drug Trade." 2021. https://www.unodc.org/southasia/frontpage/2012/october/drug-mules_-swallowed-by-the-illicit-drug-trade.html.

9. CLUB DRUGS

BBC. "Serial Killer Stephen Port Jailed for Rape Drug Murders," BBC News, November 25, 2016, https://www.bbc.com/news/uk-england-38102454.

Davis, K., and D. I. Brown. "Ketamine: Uses, Effects, Risks, and Warnings," Medical News Today, October 12, 2017, https://www.medicalnewstoday.com/articles/302663.

Dodgson, Lindsay "Middle-Class People Are Taking MDMA Wrapped in Cheese in a New Trend Called 'Brieing,'" Business Insider, May 17, 2018, https://www.businessinsider.com/posh-people-taking-mdma-with-cheese-in-brieing-trend-2018-5.

Drug Enforcement Administration. "Drug Fact Sheet: GHB." April, 2020. https://www.dea.gov/sites/default/files/2020-06/GHB-2020_0.pdf.

Drug Enforcement Administration. "Drug Fact Sheet: Rohypnol." April, 2020. https://www.dea.gov/sites/default/files/2020-06/Rohypnol-2020.pdf.

Drug Enforcement Administration. "Drug of Abuse: A DEA Resource Guide." April 24, 2020. https://www.dea.gov/sites/default/files/2020-04/Drugs%20of%20Abuse%202020-Web%20Version-508%20compliant-4-24-20_0.pdf.

Drug Enforcement Administration, Diversion Control Division, Drug and Chemical Evaluation Section. "Gamma Hydroxybutyric Acid." May 2020. https://www.deadiversion.usdoj.gov/drug_chem_info/ghb.pdf.

Drug Enforcement Administration. "Ecstasy or MDMA (Also Known as Molly)." April 2020. https://www.dea.gov/factsheets/ecstasy-or-mdma-also-known-molly.

Emergency Medical Services Association of Colorado. "Position Statement on the Safe Pre-hospitalization Use of Ketamine by EMS Professionals." November 5, 2020. https://emsac.memberclicks.net/assets/Position_Statements/Use%20of%20Ketamine%20in%20Pre-Hospital%20EMS.pdf.

Gayle, D., and C. Davies. "Alleged Serial Killer Stephen Port 'Had Appetite for Sex with Unconscious Men.'" *Guardian*, October 6, 2016. https://www.theguardian.com/uk-news/2016/oct/05/alleged-serial-killer-had-appetite-for-sex-with-unconscious-men.

Information bulletin: GHB analogs; GBL, BD, GHV, and GVL. National Drug Intelligence Center. (2002, August). Retrieved May 18, 2021, from https://www.justice.gov/archive/ndic/pubs1/1621/index.htm#Introduction.

National Drug Intelligence Center. "Information Bulletin: GHB Analogs; GBL, BD, GHV, and GVL." August 2002. https://www.justice.gov/archive/ndic/pubs1/1621/index.htm#Introduction.

National Institute on Drug Abuse. "MDMA (Ecstasy/Molly) Drug Facts." June 7, 2021. https://www.drugabuse.gov/publications/drugfacts/mdma-ecstasymolly.

National Institute on Drug Abuse. "MDMA (Ecstasy or Molly) Drug Facts, Effects." NIDA for Teens. June 25, 2021. https://teens.drugabuse.gov/drug-facts/mdma-ecstasy-or-molly#topic-5.

National Institute on Drug Abuse. "Research Report Series: MDMA (Ecstasy) Abuse." March 2006. https://www.drugabuse.gov/sites/default/files/rrmdma_0.pdf.

National Institute on Drug Abuse. "What are the effects of MDMA?" April 13, 2021. https://www.drugabuse.gov/publications/research-reports/mdma-ecstasy-abuse/what-are-effects-mdma.

Orhurhu V. J., R. Vashisht, L. E. Claus, et al. "Ketamine Toxicity." StatPearls [Internet]. Updated April 4, 2022. https://www.ncbi.nlm.nih.gov/books/NBK541087/.

Perel A., and J. T. Davidson. "Recurrent Hallucinations Following Ketamine." *Anaesthesia* 31, no. 8 (1976): 1081–83. https://doi.org/10.1111/j.1365-2044.1976.tb11948.x.

Rosenbaum S. B., V. Gupta, P. Patel, et al. "Ketamine." StatPearls [Internet]. Updated October 10, 2022. https://www.ncbi.nlm.nih.gov/books/NBK470357/.

US Food and Drug Administration. "FDA Approves New Nasal Spray Medication for Treatment-Resistant Depression; Available Only at a Certified Doctor's Office or Clinic." March 5, 2019. https://www.fda.gov/news-events/press-announcements/fda-approves-new-nasal-spray-medication-treatment-resistant-depression-available-only-certified.

Wolff, K., and A. R. Winstock. "Ketamine." *CNS Drugs* 20, no. 3 (2006): 199–218. https://doi.org/10.2165/00023210-200620030-00003.

Zandstra, P. "What Happens When You Take a Date Rape Drug Recreationally." VICE, February 8, 2018. https://tonic.vice.com/en_us/article/wjp9a4/people-are-taking-a-date-rape-drug-recreationally-and-getting-addicted.

10. HALLUCINOGENS

Albayrak, Maj E. "Microdosing: Improving Performance Enhancement in Intelligence Analysis." *Marine Corp Gazette*, February 2019. https://mca-marines.org/wp-content/uploads/Microdosing.pdf.

Antoniou, Tony, and David N. Juurlink. "Dextromethorphan Abuse." *Canadian Medical Association Journal* 186 no., 16 (2014): E631. https://doi.org/10.1503/cmaj.131676.

Associated Press. "The Latest: Oakland 2nd US City to Legalize Magic Mushrooms." June 4, 2019. https://apnews.com/article/fungi-health-drug-addiction-ca-state-wire -depression-ff023dfbf4534eba8622f504d272ff00.

Barnett, Brian S., Sloane E. Parker, and Jeremy Weleff. "United States National Institutes of Health Grant Funding for Psychedelic-Assisted Therapy Clinical Trials from 2006– 2020." *International Journal of Drug Policy* 99 (2022): 103473. https://doi.org/10.1016/j .drugpo.2021.103473.

Cespedes, Alvarao. "In the Only State Where Selling Peyote is Legal, the Cactus is Threatened and Still Controversial." *Texas Standard*, November 13, 2018. https://www.texasstandard .org/stories/in-the-only-state-where-selling-peyote-is-legal-the-cactus-is-threatened -and-still-controversial/.

Daytripnightstriper, "Life-Destroying Peyote Trip: An Experience with Peyote, MDMA, & Mushrooms," Erowid Experience Vaults, January 2, 2014, https://erowid.org /experiences/exp.php?ID=88547.

Di Marco, Marika P., David J. Edwards, Irving W. Wainer, and Murray P. Ducharme. "The Effect of Grapefruit Juice and Seville Orange Juice on the Pharmacokinetics of Dex-tromethorphan: The Role of Gut CYP3A and P-glycoprotein." *Life Sciences* 71, no. 10 (2002): 1149–60. https://doi.org/10.1016/s0024-3205(02)01799-x.

Drug Enforcement Administration; Diversion Control Division; Drug and Chemical Evalua-tion Section. "Dextromethorphan." December 2019. https://www.deadiversion.usdoj .gov/drug_chem_info/dextro_m.pdf.

Drug Enforcement Administration; Diversion Control Division; Drug and Chemical Evalua-tion Section. "D- Lysergic Acid Diethylamide." September 2019. https://www .deadiversion.usdoj.gov/drug_chem_info/lsd.pdf.

Drug Enforcement Administration. "Drug Slang Code Words." May 2017. https://www.dea. gov/sites/default/files/2018-07/DIR-020-17%20Drug%20Slang%20Code%20Words.pdf.

Drug Enforcement Administration. "DXM." April 2020. https://www.dea.gov/sites/default /files/2020-06/DXM-2020.pdf.

Drug Enforcement Administration; Department of Justice. "LSD." April 2020. https://www .dea.gov/factsheets/lsd.

Drug Enforcement Administration. "Peyote and Mescaline." April 2020. https://www.dea.gov /factsheets/peyote-and-mescaline.

Drug Enforcement Administration. "Psilocybin." April 2020. https://www.getsmartabout drugs.gov/sites/getsmartaboutdrugs.com/files/files/Psilocybin-2020.pdf.

Fuentes, Juan J., Francina Fonseca, Matilda Elices, Magi Farré, and Marta Torrens. "Therapeu-tic Use of LSD in Psychiatry: A Systematic Review of Randomized-Controlled Clinical Trials." *Frontiers in Psychiatry* 10 (2020). https://doi.org/10.3389/fpsyt.2019.00943.

Gasser, Peter, Dominique Holstein, Yvonne Michel, Rick Doblin, Berra Yazar-Klosinski, Tor-sten Passie, and Rudolf Brenneisen. "Safety and Efficacy of Lysergic Acid Diethylamide-Assisted Psychotherapy for Anxiety Associated with Life-Threatening Diseases." *Journal of Nervous & Mental Disease* 202, no. 7 (2014): 513–20. https://doi.org/10.1097/nmd .0000000000000113.

Gibson, Mary J. "This Bicycle Day, Celebrate Albert Hofmann's Psychedelic Discovery." *Roll-ing Stone*, April 19, 2020. https://www.rollingstone.com/culture/culture-news/bicycle -day-albert-hofmann-lsd-psychedelic-986279/.

Hogg, Ryan "This 'Magic' Mushroom Dispensary in Florida is Selling Psychedelics and Test-ing Legal Boundaries." *Business Insider*, October 2, 2022. https://www.businessinsider .com/magic-mushroom-dispensary-in-florida-is-testing-drug-law-boundaries-2022-10.

Hutten, Nardia, Natasha L. Mason, Patrick C. Dolder, and Kim. Kuypers. "Motives and Side-Effects of Microdosing with Psychedelics among Users." *The International Journal of Neuropsychopharmacology* 22, no. 7 (2019): 426–34. https://doi.org/10.1093/ijnp/pyz029.

Hwang, Kristine A. J., and Abdolreza Saadabadi. "Lysergic Acid Diethylamide (LSD)." StatPearls [Internet]. Updated July 11, 2022. https://www.ncbi.nlm.nih.gov/books/NBK482407/.

Journey, Jonathan D., Suneil Agrawal, and Evan. Stern. "Dextromethorphan Toxicity." StatPearls [Internet]. Updated June 25, 2020. https://www.ncbi.nlm.nih.gov/books/NBK538502/.

Kelly, J. R., M. T. Crockett, L. Alexander, M. Haran, A. Baker, L. Burke, C. Brennan, and V. O'Keane. "Psychedelic Science in Post-Covid-19 Psychiatry." *Irish Journal of Psychological Medicine* 38, no. 2 (2020): 93–98. https://doi.org/10.1017/ipm.2020.94.

Kopra, Emma I., Jason A. Ferris, James J. Rucker, Benjamin McClure, Allan H. Young, Caroline S. Copeland, and Adam R. Winstock. "Adverse Experiences Resulting in Emergency Medical Treatment Seeking Following the Use of Lysergic Acid Diethylamide (LSD)." *Journal of Psychopharmacology* 36, no. 8 (2022): 956–64. https://doi.org/10.1177/02698811221099650.

Liechti, Matthias E. "Modern Clinical Research on LSD." *Neuropsychopharmacology* 42, no. 11 (2017): 2114–27. https://doi.org/10.1038/npp.2017.86.

National Institute on Drug Abuse. "Common Hallucinogens." July 16, 2021. https://www.drugabuse.gov/publications/research-reports/hallucinogens-dissociative-drugs/what-are-dissociative-drugs.

National Institute on Drug Abuse. "How Do Hallucinogens (LSD, Psilocybin, Peyote, DMT, and Ayahuasca) Affect the Brain and Body?" June 2, 2020. https://www.drugabuse.gov/publications/research-reports/hallucinogens-dissociative-drugs/how-do-hallucinogens-lsd-psilocybin-peyote-dmt-ayahuasca-affect-brain-body.

National Institute on Drug Abuse. "N-bomb." NIDA Archives. May, 2015. https://archives.drugabuse.gov/emerging-trends/n-bomb.

NBC Universal News Group. "Father of Mind-Altering LSD Dies at 102." April 29, 2008. http://www.nbcnews.com/id/24378509/ns/technology_and_science-science/t/father-mind-altering-lsd-dies/#.XgyylUyZP2Q.

The University of Texas at Austin. "Lophophora Williamsii." Lady Bird Johnson Wildflower Center. Accessed June 3, 2021. https://www.wildflower.org/plants/result.php?id_plant=LOWI.

US Department of Agriculture. "Hallucinogens." US Forest Service. Accessed June 3, 2021. https://www.fs.usda.gov/wildflowers/ethnobotany/Mind_and_Spirit/hallucinogens.shtml.

US Department of Justice; National Drug Intelligence Center. "Psilocybin Fast Facts." Accessed August 28, 2021. https://www.justice.gov/archive/ndic/pubs6/6038/6038p.pdf.

Vohr, E. "Hopkins Scientists Show Hallucinogen in Mushrooms Creates Universal 'Mystical' Experience." Johns Hopkins Medicine. July 11, 2006. https://www.hopkinsmedicine.org/Press_releases/2006/07_11_06.html.

11. Inhalants

Baydala L. "Inhalant Abuse." *Paediatrics & Child Health* 15, no. 7 (2010): 443–54.

Centers for Disease Control and Prevention; The National Institute for Occupational Safety and Health. "Controlling Exposures to Nitrous Oxide During Anesthetic Administration." June 6, 2014. https://www.cdc.gov/niosh/docs/94-100/default.html.

Drug Science. "Alkyl Nitrites (Poppers)." March 27, 2019. http://www.drugscience.org.uk
/drugs/dissociatives/alkyl-nitrates.

National Institute on Drug Abuse; National Institutes of Health; US Department of Health
and Human Services. "Inhalants DrugFacts." April 16, 2020. https://www.drugabuse
.gov/publications/drugfacts/inhalants.

National Institute on Drug Abuse; National Institutes of Health; US Department of Health
and Human Services. "Research Report Series: Inhalants." July 2012. https://
d14rmgtrwzf5a.cloudfront.net/sites/default/files/inhalantsrrs.pdf.

Pfizer Labs. "Viagra (sildenafil citrate)." March 2014. https://www.accessdata.fda.gov
/drugsatfda_docs/label/2014/20895s039s042lbl.pdf.

SNOHOMISH County Health District Bulletin. "Street or Slang Names for Drugs." 2019. Accessed August 1, 2021. https://www.snohd.org/DocumentCenter/View/2516/Drug
_Names_Slang_2019_05_09?bidId=.

US Food and Drug Administration. "Ingesting or Inhaling Nitrite 'Poppers' Can Cause Severe
Injury or Death." July 15, 2021. https://www.fda.gov/consumers/consumer-updates
/nitrite-poppers.

Williams, Janet F., and Michael Storck. "Inhalant Abuse." *Pediatrics* 119, no. 5 (2007): 1009–17.
https://doi.org/10.1542/peds.2007-0470.

12. Leafy Leftovers

American Association of Poison Control Centers. "Synthetic Cannabinoids." August 2021.
https://aapcc.org/track/synthetic-cannabinoids.

Berdai, Mohamed A., Smael Labib, Khadija Chetouani, and Mustapha Harandou. "Atropa Belladonna Intoxication: A Case Report." *The Pan African Medical Journal* 11, no. 72 (2012).

Bush, Donna, and David Woodwell. "Update: Drug-Related Emergency Department Visits
Involving Synthetic Cannabinoids." *CBHSQ Report*, October 16, 2014. https://www
.samhsa.gov/data/sites/default/files/Update%20%20Drug-Related%20Emergency
%20Department%20Visits%20Involving%20Synthetic%20Cannabinoids/Update
%20%20Drug-Related%20Emergency%20Department%20Visits%20Involving
%20Synthetic%20Cannabinoids.htm.

Cash, Mary C., Katherine Cunnane, Chuyin Fan, and E. Alfonso Romero-Sandoval. (2020).
"Mapping Cannabis Potency in Medical and Recreational Programs in the United
States." *PLOS ONE* 15, no. 3 (2020). https://doi.org/10.1371/journal.pone.0230167.

Centers for Disease Control and Prevention. "Outbreak Alert Update: Potential Life-Threatening Vitamin K-Dependent Antagonist Coagulopathy Associated with Synthetic Cannabinoids Use." April 23, 2018. https://emergency.cdc.gov/newsletters/coca/042318
.html.

Centers for Disease Control and Prevention. "Synthetic Cannabinoids: An Overview for
Healthcare Providers." April 24, 2018. https://www.cdc.gov/nceh/hsb/chemicals/sc
/healthcare.html.

Chadwick, Andrew, Abigail Ash, James Day, and Mark Borthwick. "Accidental Overdose in
the Deep Shade of Night: A Warning on the Assumed Safety of 'Natural Substances.'"
BMJ Case Reports (2015). https://doi.org/10.1136/bcr-2015-209333.

Collins, Suzanne. *The Hunger Games*. New York: Scholastic, 2010.

Cutlip, Hunter A., Ella Bushman, Lisa Thottumari, Roja Mogallapu, and Michael Ang-Ra-
banes. "A Case Report of Kratom-Induced Psychosis." *Cureus* (2021). https://doi
.org/10.7759/cureus.16073.

Davies M. K., and A. Hollman. "Atropa Belladonna." *Heart*. 88, no. 3 (2002): 215. https://doi
.org/10.1136/heart.88.3.215-a.

Dawson, Andrew H., and Nichols A. Buckley. "Pharmacological Management of Anticholinergic Delirium—Theory, Evidence and Practice." *British Journal of Clinical Pharmacology* 81, no. 3 (2016): 516–24. https://doi.org/10.1111/bcp.12839.

Drug Enforcement Administration. "The Facts about Marijuana Concentrates." Get the Facts about Drugs: Just Think Twice. Accessed June 2021. https://www.justthinktwice.gov /facts-about-marijuana-concentrates.

Drug Enforcement Administration; U.S. Department of Justice. "Drug of Abuse: A DEA Resource Guide." (2020). https://www.dea.gov/sites/default/files/2020-04/Drugs %20of%20Abuse%202020-Web%20Version-508%20compliant-4-24-20_0.pdf.

Editors of Encyclopedia Britannica. "Belladonna." *Encyclopedia Britannica.* May 17, 2017. https://www.britannica.com/plant/belladonna.

European Agency for the Evaluation of Medicinal Products: Veterinary Medicine Evaluation Unit. "Atropa Belladonna Summary Report." December 1998. https://www.ema.europa .eu/en/documents/mrl-report/atropa-belladonna-summary-report-committee -veterinary-medicinal-products_en.pdf.

Food and Drug Administration. "FDA and Cannabis: Research and Drug Approval Process." October 2022. https://www.fda.gov/news-events/public-health-focus/fda-and -cannabis-research-and-drug-approval-process.

Food and Drug Administration. "FDA and Kratom." April 27, 2022. https://www.fda.gov/news -events/public-health-focus/fda-and-kratom.

Food and Drug Administration. "FDA Announces Seizure of Adulterated Dietary Supplements Containing Kratom." May 2021. https://www.fda.gov/news-events/press -announcements/fda-announces-seizure-adulterated-dietary-supplements-containing -kratom.

Food and Drug Administration. "FDA Approves New Indication for Drug Containing an Active Ingredient Derived from Cannabis to Treat Seizures in Rare Genetic Disease." July 31, 2020. https://www.fda.gov/news-events/press-announcements/fda-approves-new -indication-drug-containing-active-ingredient-derived-cannabis-treat-seizures-rare.

Food and Drug Administration. "FDA Orders Mandatory Recall for Kratom Products Due to Risk of Salmonella." April 2018. https://www.fda.gov/news-events/press -announcements/fda-orders-mandatory-recall-kratom-products-due-risk-salmonella.

Food and Drug Administration. "FDA Warns Companies Illegally Selling Over-the-Counter CBD Products for Pain Relief." March 2021. https://www.fda.gov/news-events/press -announcements/fda-warns-companies-illegally-selling-over-counter-cbd-products -pain-relief.

Food and Drug Administration. "FDA Warns Consumers about Homeopathic Teething Products." November 2019. https://www.fda.gov/drugs/information-drug-class/fda-warns -consumers-about-homeopathic-teething-products.

Food and Drug Administration. "Statement from FDA Commissioner Scott Gottlieb, M.D. on FDA Advisory about Deadly Risks Associated with Kratom." April 2018. https://www .fda.gov/news-events/press-announcements/statement-fda-commissioner-scott -gottlieb-md-fda-advisory-about-deadly-risks-associated-kratom.

Gerald Gianutsos, P. D. "The DEA Changes Its Mind on Kratom." US Pharmacist—The Leading Journal in Pharmacy. March 17, 2017. https://www.uspharmacist.com/article/the -dea-changes-its-mind-on-kratom.

Havenon, A. de, B. Chin, K. C. Thomas, and P. Afra. "The Secret 'Spice': An Undetectable Toxic Cause of Seizure." *The Neurohospitalist* 1, no. 4 (2011): 182–86. https://doi.org/10 .1177/1941874411417977.

Jackson, M. "'Divine Stramonium': The Rise and Fall of Smoking for Asthma." *Medical History* 54, no. 2 (2011): 171–94. https://doi.org/10.1017/s0025727300000235.

Keeler, M. H., and F. J. Kane. "The Use of Hyoscyamine as a Hallucinogen and Intoxicant." *American Journal of Psychiatry* 124, no. 6 (2006): 852–54. https://doi.org/10.1176/ajp .124.6.852.

Kratom.org. "A Detailed Guide to the 'Toss & Wash' Method." February 1, 2022. https:// kratom.org/guides/how-to-take-kratom/toss-and-wash/.

Macleod, N. "The Bromide Sleep: A New Departure in the Treatment of Acute Mania." *BMJ* 1, no. 2038 (1900): 134–36. https://doi.org/10.1136/bmj.1.2038.134.

Meier, M. H., A. Caspi, A. Ambler, H. Harrington, R. Houts, R. S. Keefe, K. McDonald, A. Ward, R. Poulton, and T. E. Moffitt. "Persistent Cannabis Users Show Neuropsychological Decline from Childhood to Midlife." *Proceedings of the National Academy of Sciences* 109, no. 40 (2012): E2657–E2664. https://doi.org/10.1073/pnas.1206820109.

National Center for Biotechnology Information. "PubChem Compound Summary for CID 154417, Hyoscyamine." *PubChem* (2022). https://pubchem.ncbi.nlm.nih.gov/compound /Hyoscyamine.

National Institute on Drug Abuse. "Kratom DrugFacts." April 2019. https://www.drugabuse .gov/publications/drugfacts/kratom.

National Institute on Drug Abuse. "Marijuana (Weed, Cannabis) Drug Facts, Effects." July 16, 2021. NIDA for Teens. https://teens.drugabuse.gov/drug-facts/marijuana.

National Institute on Drug Abuse; National Institutes of Health; US Department of Health and Human Services. "Marijuana DrugFacts." December 2019. https://www.drugabuse .gov/publications/drugfacts/marijuana.

National Institute on Drug Addiction; National Institutes of Health; US Department of Health and Human Services. "Spice." NIDA for Teens. June 25, 2021. https://teens .drugabuse.gov/drug-facts/spice.

National Institute on Drug Abuse; National Institutes of Health; US Department of Health and Human Services. "Synthetic Cannabinoids (K2/Spice) DrugFacts." February 5, 2018. https://www.drugabuse.gov/publications/drugfacts/synthetic-cannabinoids -k2spice.

Neerman M. F., R. E. Frost, and J. Deking. "A Drug Fatality Involving Kratom." *Journal of Forensic Science* 58, no. s1 (January 2013): S278–S279. https://doi.org/10.1111/1556 -4029.12009.

Olsen, E. O. M., J. O'Donnell, C. L. Mattson, J. G. Schier, and N. Wilson. "Notes from the Field: Unintentional Drug Overdose Deaths with Kratom Detected—27 States, July 2016–December 2017." *MMWR. Morbidity and Mortality Weekly Report* 68, no. 14 (2019): 326–27. https://doi.org/10.15585/mmwr.mm6814a2.

Post S., H. A. Spiller, T. Chounthirath, G. A. Smith. "Kratom Exposures Reported to United States Poison Control Centers: 2011–2017." *Clinical Toxicology* 57, no. 10 (October 2019): 847–54. https://doi.org/10.1080/15563650.2019.1569236.

Shakespeare, William. *The Tragedy of Macbeth.* Edited by George Lyman Kittredge. New York: Wiley, 1996.

Swogger, M. T., K. E. Smith, A. Garcia-Romeu, O. Grundmann, C. A. Veltri, J. Henningfield, and L. Y. Busch. "Understanding Kratom Use: A Guide for Healthcare Providers." *Frontiers in Pharmacology* 13 (2022). https://doi.org/10.3389/fphar.2022.801855.

US Forest Service. "The Powerful Solanaceae: Belladonna." Accessed June 17, 2021. https:// www.fs.usda.gov/wildflowers/ethnobotany/Mind_and_Spirit/belladonna.shtml.

13. Opioids

Abi-Aad, Karl R., and Armen Derian. "Hydromorphone." StatPearls [Internet]. Updated July 11, 2022. https://www.ncbi.nlm.nih.gov/books/NBK470393/.

Ball, Laura J., Colin Venner, Rommel G. Tirona, Eric Arts, Kaveri Gupta, Joshua C. Wiener, Sharon Koivu, and Michael S. Silverman. "Heating Injection Drug Preparation Equipment Used for Opioid Injection May Reduce HIV Transmission Associated with Sharing Equipment." *JAIDS Journal of Acquired Immune Deficiency Syndromes* 81, no. 4 (2019). https://doi.org/10.1097/qai.0000000000002063.

Centers for Disease Control and Prevention. "Drug Overdose Deaths Remain High." March 3, 2021. https://www.cdc.gov/drugoverdose/deaths/index.html.

Centers for Disease Control and Prevention. "Fentanyl." February 16, 2021. https://www.cdc.gov/opioids/basics/fentanyl.html.

Centers for Disease Control and Prevention. "Influx of Fentanyl-Laced Counterfeit Pills and Toxic Fentanyl-Related Compounds Further Increases Risk of Fentanyl-Related Overdose and Fatalities." August 15, 2016. https://emergency.cdc.gov/han/han00395.asp.

Centers for Disease Control and Prevention. "Synthetic Opioid Overdose Data." March 25, 2021. https://www.cdc.gov/drugoverdose/deaths/synthetic/index.html.

Centers for Disease Control and Prevention. "Vital Signs: Demographic and Substance Use Trends among Heroin Users—United States, 2002–2013." July 10, 2015. https://www.cdc.gov/mmwr/preview/mmwrhtml/mm6426a3.htm.

Chowdhury, Mursheda M., and Richard Board. "Morphine-Induced Hallucinations—Resolution with Switching to Oxycodone: A Case Report and Review of the Literature." *Cases Journal* 2, no. 9391 (December 2009). https://doi.org/10.1186/1757-1626-2-9391.

Drug Enforcement Administration. "Opium." April 2020. https://www.dea.gov/factsheets/opium.

Drug Enforcement Administration; Office of Intelligence. "Opium Poppy Cultivation and Heroin Processing in Southeast Asia." September 1992. https://www.ojp.gov/pdffiles1/Digitization/141189NCJRS.pdf.

Drug Enforcement Administration. "Oxycodone." January 2023. https://www.deadiversion.usdoj.gov/drug_chem_info/oxycodone.pdf.

Drug Enforcement Administration; Diversion Control Division; Drug and Chemical Evaluation Section. "Desomorphine." December 2019. https://www.deadiversion.usdoj.gov/drug_chem_info/desomorphine.pdf.

Drug Enforcement Administration; Diversion Control Division; Drug and Chemical Evaluation Section. "Unwashed Poppy Seeds." November 2019. https://www.deadiversion.usdoj.gov/drug_chem_info/unwashed_poppy_seed.pdf.

Drug Enforcement Administration. "Drug Enforcement Agency Announces the Seizure of Over 379 Million Deadly Doses of Fentanyl in 2022." https://www.dea.gov/press-releases/2022/12/20/drug-enforcement-administration-announces-seizure-over-379-million-deadly.

Durrani, Mehnoor, and Kamna Bansal. "Methadone." Updated February 12, 2022. StatPearls [Internet]. https://www.ncbi.nlm.nih.gov/books/NBK562216/.

Erowid. "Heroin Basics." Erowid Heroin Vault: Basics. Accessed May 2020. https://erowid.org/chemicals/heroin/heroin_basics.shtml.

Food and Drug Administration. "FDA Requires Labeling Changes for Prescription Opioid Cough and Cold Medicines to Limit Their Use To Adults 18 Years and Older." January 11, 2018. https://www.fda.gov/drugs/drug-safety-and-availability/fda-drug-safety-communication-fda-requires-labeling-changes-prescription-opioid-cough-and-cold.

Food and Drug Administration. "FDA Restricts Use of Prescription Codeine Pain and Cough Medicines and Tramadol Pain Medicines in Children; Recommends against Use in Breastfeeding Women. April 2017. https://www.fda.gov/Drugs/DrugSafety/ucm549679.htm.

Hatch-Maillette, Mary A., K. Michelle Peavy, Judith I. Tsui, Caleb J. Banta-Green, Stephen Woolworth, and Paul Grekin. "Re-thinking Patient Stability for Methadone in Opioid Treatment Programs during a Global Pandemic: Provider Perspectives." *Journal of Substance Abuse Treatment* 124 (2021). https://doi.org/10.1016/j.jsat.2020.108223.

Health and Human Services. "Opioid Facts and Statistics" HHS.gov. Accessed April 8, 2021. https://www.hhs.gov/opioids/statistics/index.html.

Huecker, Martin R., George A. Koutsothanasis, Muhammed S. U. Abbasy MSU, et al. "Heroin." Updated September 9, 2022. StatPearls [Internet]. https://www.ncbi.nlm.nih.gov/books/NBK441876/.

Jones, Christopher M., Grant T. Baldwin, Teresa Manocchio, Jessica O. White, and Karin A. Mack. "Trends in Methadone Distribution for Pain Treatment, Methadone Diversion, and Overdose Deaths-United States, 2002–2014." *MMWR Morb Mortal Wkly Rep* 65 (2016):667–71.

McCarty, Dennis, Christina Bougatsos, Brian Chan, Kim A. Hoffman, Kelsey C. Priest, Sara Grusing, and Roger Chou. "Office-Based Methadone Treatment for Opioid Use Disorder and Pharmacy Dispensing: A Scoping Review." *American Journal of Psychiatry* 178, no. 9 (2021): 804–17. https://doi.org/10.1176/appi.ajp.2021.20101548.

Moss, Michael J., Brandon J. Warrick, Lewis S. Nelson, Charles A. McKay, Pierre-André Dubé, Sophie Gosselin, Robert B. Palmer, and Andrew I. Stolbach. "ACMT and AACT Position Statement: Preventing Occupational Fentanyl and Fentanyl Analog Exposure to Emergency Responders." *Clin Toxicol (Phila).* 56, no.4 (2018):297–300. https://doi: 10.1080/15563650.2017.1373782.

National Institute on Drug Abuse. "Heroin Use Is Rare in Prescription Drug Users." April 13, 2021. https://www.drugabuse.gov/publications/research-reports/prescription-opioids-heroin/heroin-use-rare-in-prescription-drug-users.

National Institute on Drug Abuse. "Krokodil." May 2015. National Institute on Drug Abuse Archives. https://archives.drugabuse.gov/emerging-trends/krokodil.

National Institute on Drug Abuse. "Nearly Half of Opioid-Related Overdose Deaths Involve Fentanyl." June 12, 2020. https://www.drugabuse.gov/news-events/news-releases/2018/05/nearly-half-of-opioid-related-overdose-deaths-involve-fentanyl.

National Institute on Drug Abuse. "Opioid Exposure Associated with Poppy Consumption Reported to Poison Control Centers and the US Food and Drug Administration." March 25, 2021. https://www.drugabuse.gov/news-events/emerging-trend/opioid-exposure-associated-poppy-consumption-reported-to-poison-control-centers-us-food-drug.

National Institute on Drug Abuse. "Prescription Opioid and Heroin Research Report: Introduction." August 3, 2021. https://www.drugabuse.gov/publications/research-reports/prescription-opioids-heroin/introduction.

National Institute on Drug Abuse. "What Is the Scope of Heroin Use in the United States?" April 13, 2021. https://www.drugabuse.gov/publications/research-reports/heroin/scope-heroin-use-in-united-states.

National Institute on Drug Abuse; National Institutes of Health; US Department of Health and Human Services. "Fentanyl Drug Facts." June 2021. https://www.drugabuse.gov/drug-topics/fentanyl.

National Institute on Drug Abuse; National Institutes of Health; US Department of Health and Human Services. "Heroin." July 16, 2021. https://teens.drugabuse.gov/drug-facts /heroin.

National Institute on Drug Abuse; National Institutes of Health; US Department of Health and Human Services. "Heroin DrugFacts." June 2021. https://www.drugabuse.gov /publications/drugfacts/heroin.

Oelhaf, Robert C., and Mohammadreza Azadfard. "Heroin Toxicity." Updated May 15, 2022. StatPearls [Internet]. https://www.ncbi.nlm.nih.gov/books/NBK430736/.

Public Health Service, HHS. "Title 42: Part 8 Medication Assisted Treatment for Opioid Use Disorders." November 2022. https://www.ecfr.gov/current/title-42/chapter-I /subchapter-A/part-8.

Riches, James R., Robert W. Read, Robin M. Black, Nichols J. Cooper, and Christopher M. Timperley. "Analysis of Clothing and Urine from Moscow Theatre Siege Casualties Reveals Carfentanil and Remifentanil Use." *Journal of Analytical Toxicology* 36, no. 9 (2012): 647–56. https://doi.org/10.1093/jat/bks078.

Rosenblum, Andrew, Lisa A. Marsch, Herman Joseph, and Russell K. Portenoy. "Opioids and the Treatment of Chronic Pain: Controversies, Current Status, and Future Directions." *Experimental and Clinical Psychopharmacology* 16, no. 5 (2008): 405–16. https://doi.org /10.1037/a0013628.

Samano, Kimberly L., Randall E. Clouette, Barbara J. Rowland, and R. H. Barry Sample. "Concentrations of Morphine and Codeine in Paired Oral Fluid and Urine Specimens Following Ingestion of a Poppy Seed Roll and Raw Poppy Seeds." *J Anal Toxicol.* 39, no.8 (2015): 655–61. https://doi: 10.1093/jat/bkv081.

UN Office on Drugs and Crime. "Bulletin on Narcotics." No. 2–003. (January 1953). https:// www.unodc.org/unodc/en/data-and-analysis/bulletin/bulletin_1953-01-01_2 _page004.html#bf031.

US Department of Justice; Drug Intelligence Office. OxyContin Fast Facts. https://www .justice.gov/archive/ndic/pubs6/6025/6025p.pdf.

US National Library of Medicine. "Morphine." *MedlinePlus.* February 2021. https:// medlineplus.gov/druginfo/meds/a682133.html.

Whelan, Paul J., and Kimberly Remski. "Buprenorphine vs. Methadone Treatment: A Review of Evidence in Both Developed and Developing Worlds." *J Neurosci Rural Pract* 3, no.1 (2012): 45–50. https://doi:10.4103/0976-3147.91934.

14. SEDATIVES

American Addiction Centers. "Valium Facts, History and Statistics." DrugAbuse.com. August 20, 2021. https://drugabuse.com/benzodiazepines/valium/history-and-statistics/.

Crowhurst, J. A. "The Historical Significance of Anaesthesia Events at Pearl Harbor." *Anaesthesia and Intensive Care* 42, no. 1(2014): 21–24. https://doi.org/10.1177 /0310057X1404201S03.

Death Penalty Information Center. "FDA Issues Final Order Refusing to Release Illegally Imported Lethal-Injection Drugs to States." April 24, 2017. https://deathpenaltyinfo.org /news/fda-issues-final-order-refusing-to-release-illegally-imported-lethal-injection -drugs-to-states.

Drug Enforcement Administration. "Barbiturates." April 2020. https://www.getsmartabout drugs.gov/sites/getsmartaboutdrugs.com/files/files/Barbiturates-2020.pdf.

Drug Enforcement Administration. "Drugs of Abuse: A DEA Resource Guide." 2020. https:// www.dea.gov/sites/default/files/2020-04/Drugs%20of%20Abuse%202020-Web %20Version-508%20compliant-4-24-20_0.pdf.

Environmental Protection Agency. "Chloroform." January 2020. https://www.epa.gov/sites /default/files/2016-09/documents/chloroform.pdf.

Erland Lauren A., and Praveen K. Saxena. "Melatonin Natural Health Products and Supplements: Presence of Serotonin and Significant Variability of Melatonin Content." *Journal of Clinial Sleep Medicine* 13, no. 2 (February 2017): 275–81. https://doi.org/10.5664/jcsm .6462.

Food and Drug Administration. "FDA Drug Safety Communication: FDA Warns about Serious Risks and Death When Combining Opioid Pain or Cough Medicines with Benzodiazepines; Requires Its Strongest Warning." September 20, 2017. https://www .fda.gov/drugs/drug-safety-and-availability/fda-drug-safety-communication-fda-warns -about-serious-risks-and-death-when-combining-opioid-pain-or.

Foxall, K. "Chloroform Toxicological Overview." Health Protection Agency Center for Radiation, Chemical and Environmental Hazards. 2007. https://assets.publishing.service.gov .uk/government/uploads/system/uploads/attachment_data/file/338535/Chloroform _Toxicological_Overview.pdf.

Greenberg, Michael I. "Benzodiazepine Withdrawal." *Emergency Medicine News* 23, no. 12 (2001): 18. https://doi.org/10.1097/01.eem.0000292622.83311.c3.

Grissinger Matthew "Chloral Hydrate: Is It Still Being Used? Are There Safer Alternatives?" 2019. https://www.ncbi.nlm.nih.gov/pmc/articles/PMC6679948/.

Health and Human Services. "Melatonin: What You Need to Know." National Center for Complementary and Integrative Health. July 2022. https://www.nccih.nih.gov/health /melatonin-what-you-need-to-know.

Institute for Safe Medication Practices. "Chloral Hydrate: Is It Still Being Used? Are There Safer Alternatives?" November 3, 2016. https://www.ismp.org/resources/chloral -hydrate-it-still-being-used-are-there-safer-alternatives.

Kang Michael, Michael A. Galuska, and Sassan Ghassemzadeh. "Benzodiazepine Toxicity." StatPearls [Internet]. Updated June 27, 2022. https://www.ncbi.nlm.nih.gov/books /NBK482238/.

Lelak, Karima, Varun Vohra, Mark I. Neuman, Michael S. Toce, and Usha Sethuraman. "Pediatric Melatonin Ingestions—United States, 2012–2021." *MMWR. Morbidity and Mortality Weekly Report* 71, no. 22 (2022): 725–29. https://doi.org/10.15585/mmwr.mm7122a1.

López-Muñoz, Francisco, Ronaldo Ucha-Udabe, and Cecilio Alamo. "The History of Barbiturates a Century after Their Clinical Introduction." *Neuropsychiatric Disease and Treatment* 1, no. 4 (2005): 329–43.

Macleod, Neil "The Bromide Sleep: A New Departure in the Treatment of Acute Mania." *BMJ* 1, no. 2038 (1900): 134–36. https://doi.org/10.1136/bmj.1.2038.134.

Mayer, L. D., and I. Greenfield. "Barbiturate Poisoning." *Archives of Internal Medicine* 84, no. 3 (1949): 379. https://doi.org/10.1001/archinte.1949.00230030021002.

Merkel, Howard "The Day Judy Garland's Star Burned Out." PBS Newshour. June 29, 2019. https://www.pbs.org/newshour/health/the-day-judy-garlands-star-burned-out #:~:text=Her%20husband%20of%20only%20three,still%20holding%20up%20her %20head.

Roth, Veronica. *Insurgent*. New York: Harper Collins, 2012.

Suddock, Jolee T., and Matthew D. Cain. "Barbiturate Toxicity." StatPearls [Internet]. Updated July 2, 2020. https://www.ncbi.nlm.nih.gov/books/NBK499875/.

Tordjman, Sylvie, Sylvie Chokron, Richard Delorme, Amaëlle Charrier, Eric Bellissant, Namat Jaafari, and Claire Fougerou. "Melatonin: Pharmacology, Functions and Therapeutic Benefits." *Current Neuropharmacology* 15, no. 3 (April 2017): 434–43. https://doi.org/10.2174/1570159X14666161228122115.

Yamamoto, T., P. I. Dargan, A. Dines, C. Yates, F. Heyerdahl, K. E. Hovda, I. Giraudon, R. Sedefov, and D. M. Wood. "Concurrent Use of Benzodiazepine by Heroin Users—What Are the Prevalence and the Risks Associated with This Pattern of Use?" *Journal of Medical Toxicology* 15, no. 1 (2019): 4–11. https://doi.org/10.1007/s13181-018-0674-4.

15. Stimulants

Auten, Jonathan D., and Michael J. Matteucci. "Methamphetamine Poisoning." California Poison Control System (CPCS). September 20, 2008. https://calpoison.org/news/methamphetamine-poisoning.

Branum, Amy M., Lauren M. Rossen, and Kenneth C. Schoendorf. "Trends in Caffeine Intake among Us Children and Adolescents." *Pediatrics* 133, no. 3 (2014): 386–93. https://doi.org/10.1542/peds.2013-2877.

Butte County Sheriff's Office. "Meth Facts." Butte County. Accessed September 2021. http://www.buttecounty.net/sheriffcoroner/methfacts.

Cappelletti, Simone, Daria Piacentino, Vittorio Fineschi, Paola Frati, Luigi Cipolloni, and Mariarosaria Aromatario. "Caffeine-Related Deaths: Manner of Deaths and Categories at Risk." *Nutrients* 10, no. 5 (2018): 611. https://doi.org/10.3390/nu10050611.

Centers for Disease Control and Prevention. "Alcohol and Caffeine." February 4, 2020. https://www.cdc.gov/alcohol/fact-sheets/caffeine-and-alcohol.htm.

Centers for Disease Control and Prevention; CDC Healthy Schools. (2019, May 29). "The Buzz on Energy Drinks." May 29, 2019. https://www.cdc.gov/healthyschools/nutrition/energy.htm.

Drug Enforcement Administration. "Amphetamines." April 2020. https://www.dea.gov/factsheets/amphetamines.

Drug Enforcement Administration. "Cocaine." April 2020. https://www.dea.gov/factsheets/cocaine.

Drug Enforcement Administration. "Drugs of Abuse: A DEA Resource Guide." 2020. https://www.dea.gov/sites/default/files/2020-04/Drugs%20of%20Abuse%202020-Web%20Version-508%20compliant-4-24-20_0.pdf.

Duke University. "Content Background: Why is Smoked Cocaine (Crack) More Likely to be Abused or Addictive Than Snorted Cocaine?" Pharmacology Education Partnership. 2013. https://sites.duke.edu/thepepproject/module-1-acids-bases-and-cocaine-addicts/content-background-why-is-smoked-cocaine-crack-more-likely-to-be-abused-or-addictive-than-snorted-cocaine/.

Duncan, Allison, and David Dixon. "Presentation of Caffeine Intoxication in an Active Duty Service Member Originally Believed to Have a Psychotic Disorder." *Cureus*, (2021). https://doi.org/10.7759/cureus.18615.

Food and Drug Administration. "Caffeinated Alcoholic Beverages." November 17, 2010. https://www.fda.gov/food/food-additives-petitions/caffeinated-alcoholic-beverages.

Food and Drug Administration. "FDA Warns Consumers about Pure and Highly Concentrated Caffeine." April 2018. https://www.fda.gov/food/dietary-supplement-products-ingredients/fda-warns-consumers-about-pure-and-highly-concentrated-caffeine#:~:text=What%20to%20do,dangerous%20or%20even%20lethal%20amount.

Evans Justin, John R. Richards, and Amanda S. Battisti. "Caffeine." StatPearls [Internet]. Updated May 1, 2022. https://www.ncbi.nlm.nih.gov/books/NBK519490/.

Forrester, J. M., A. W. Steele, J. A. Waldron, and P. E. Parsons. "Crack Lung: An Acute Pulmonary Syndrome with a Spectrum of Clinical and Histopathologic Findings." *American Review of Respiratory Disease* 142, no. 2 (1990): 462–67. https://doi.org/10.1164/ajrccm /142.2.462.

Hearn, John K., Thea Reiff, Anne B. McBride, and Michael B. Kelly. (2020). "Caffeine-Induced Psychosis and a Review of the Statutory Approaches to Involuntary Intoxication." *Journal of the American Academy of Psychiatry and the Law* 48, no. 3 (2020): 376–83. https:// pubmed.ncbi.nlm.nih.gov/32404360/.

Karch, Steven B. "Cocaine: History, Use, Abuse." *Journal of the Royal Society of Medicine* 92, no. 8 (1999): 393–97. https://doi.org/10.1177/014107689909200803.

Kon, O. M., J. B. Redhead, D. Gillen, J. Fothergill, J. A. Henry, and D. M. Mitchell. "'Crack Lung' Caused by an Impure Preparation." *Thorax* 51, no. 9 (1996): 959–60. https://doi .org/10.1136/thx.51.9.959.

Library of Congress. "Cocaine Crisis (1898–1915): Topics in Chronicling America." Research Guides. Accessed September 2020. https://guides.loc.gov/chronicling-america-cocaine.

Morton W. Alexander, and Gwendolyn G. Stockton. "Methylphenidate Abuse and Psychiatric Side Effects." *Primary Care Companion to the Journal of Clinical Psychiatry* 2, no. 5 (2000): 159–64. https://doi.org/10.4088/pcc.v02n0502.

National Institute on Drug Abuse. "Is Caffeine Really Addictive?" May 10, 2016. https:// archives.drugabuse.gov/blog/post/caffeine-really-addictive.

National Institute on Drug Abuse; National Institutes of Health; US Department of Health and Human Services. "Methamphetamine DrugFacts." May 16, 2019. https://www .drugabuse.gov/publications/drugfacts/methamphetamine.

National Institute on Drug Abuse; National Institutes of Health; US Department of Health and Human Services. "Prescription Stimulants DrugFacts." June 2018. https://www .drugabuse.gov/publications/drugfacts/prescription-stimulants.

Recordati Rare Diseases, Inc. "Desoxyn (Methamphetamine Hydrochloride Tablets, USP) Package Insert." Food and Drug Administration. 2017. https://www.accessdata.fda.gov /drugsatfda_docs/label/2017/005378s034lbl.pdf.

US Department of Justice; Drug Enforcement Administration. "2020 National Drug Threat Assessment." March 2021. https://www.dea.gov/sites/default/files/2021-02/DIR-008 -21%202020%20National%20Drug%20Threat%20Assessment_WEB.pdf.

Viner, Kendra "Cluster of Cocaine-Fentanyl Overdoses in Philadelphia Underscores Need for More 'Test Strips' and Rapid Response." *Penn Medicine News*, November 1, 2018. https:// www.pennmedicine.org/news/news-releases/2018/november/cocaine-fentanyl -overdoses-in-philadelphia-need-more-test-strips-and-rapid-response.

INDEX

acetaminophen, 89; in combination medications, 124–25, 156, 168; overdose, 171

acid, LSD, 49, 57, 68–71, 77, 82; battery, 70; blotter, 70; hydrochloric, 147

acid reflux, 188

Adderall, 12, 189, 199; combined with caffeine, 187; combined with GHB, 64; counterfeit, 39, 129–30, 200

addiction: Adderall, 208; barbiturates, 2, 176; bath salts, 42; benzodiazepine, 177; caffeine, 186; fentanyl, 131–33; GHB, 65; hallucinogen, 68; hallucinogenic mushrooms, 81; heroin, 138, 140–41; hydromorphone, 143; inhalants, 99; kratom, 109; krokodil, 147; LSD, 73; methamphetamine, 185, 200, 204–5; morphine, 156–57, 165; opioid, 2; opium, 163–64; oxycodone, 169; z-drugs, 178

addiction, treatment of: LSD, 69, 75; hallucinogenic mushrooms, 76; mescaline, 82; methadone, 150–52

Addys, 4, 207, 209

ADHD (attention deficit hyperactivity disorder), 199, 200, 207–10

adrenaline surges, bath salts, 38, 42

aggressive behavior: amphetamines, 211; bath salts, 42–43; cocaine, 196; GHB, 65; methamphetamine, 203–6

aggressive behavior treated with ketamine, 57

agitation, 12–14; amphetamines, 209, 211; antihistamines, 33; barbiturate withdrawal, 181; bath salts, 40, 43; belladonna, 104, 107; benzodiazepine withdrawal, 182; caffeine, 188; cocaine, 53, 194–97; dextromethorphan

(DXM), 91; kratom, 109; marijuana withdrawal, 118; methamphetamine, 203, 206; NBOMe, 70; Spice/K2, 121

alcohol, 20–29, 31; baths, 20–21, 24; blood level, 25; caffeine, 186; enemas, 22, 24, 26–27; Jell-O shots, 23–25; methanol, 23–24; poisoning, 21–23; rubbing alcohol, 20–21, 24, 26; tampons, 21–22, 24–27; vaping, 22–23, 25, 27

alcohol combined with: barbiturates, 176–77; ketamine, 57, 59; methadone, 153–54; roofies, 54–55

alertness, 185, 187–88, 197–98, 207

alprazolam, 11, 177, 179; counterfeit, 129

Ambien, 178

amitriptyline, 29

amnesia, 11, 49, 53, 63, 66, 176–77, 181

amobarbital, 175–76, 179

amphetamines, 12, 59, 199; methamphetamine, 198–206; prescription, 206–12

amyl nitrite (poppers), 95–101

amys, 62, 96, 228

anesthetic, 56, 96, 175, 190, 193, 218, 226

antidepressants, 13, 29–31, 90; with dextromethorphan (DXM), 88, 90

antihistamines, 13, 33–37; Blue velvet, 166; combined with codeine, 124; combined with dextromethorphan (DXM), 89

anxiety, 11, 90, 83; amphetamines, 208; barbiturate withdrawal, 18; benzodiazepines, 177, 180; benzodiazepine withdrawal, 182; bromides, 2; chloral hydrate, 2; ecstasy, 52; GHB withdrawal, 65; hallucinogenic

smoke by vape: alcohol, 24, 26–28; marijuana, 115; THC concentrates, 112–13, 116–18; Spice/K2, 121. *See also* smoke

snort: alcohol, 21–22, 24; bath salts, 40–14, 43; benzodiazepines, 180; cocaine, 190, 192–97; ecstasy, 50–51; fentanyl, 133, 136; GHB, 64; heroin, 138–142; hydromorphone, 143–46; ketamine, 59, 61; methamphetamine, 201–2, 205–6; morphine, 160–62; oxycodone, 168, 170–72; prescription stimulants, 208–09, 211–12; roofies, 54; Suboxone, 152; tranq dope, 135

Special K, 58

speech, garbled by antihistamines, 35

speech, slurred, 10–11; alcohol, 25; dextromethorphan (DXM), 91; inhalants, 98; ketamine, 60–61; roofies, 55

speedballing, 139, 194, 201

Spice/K2, 12, 14, 102, 119–23; in bath salts, 38

sprays, nasal: benzodiazepine, 180, 183; fentanyl, 133; ketamine, 58–61; naloxone, 17

SSRI, 29, 31

stacking, 78

stamps, 71

stimulants, 12; bath salts, 39–40; caffeine, 185–90; cocaine, 190–198; dextromethorphan (DXM), 91; kratom, 108; methamphetamine, 198–206; prescription stimulants, 200, 206–12; speedball, 139

street supplies: bath salts, 39; cocaine, 197; drug shortage impact on, 209; fentanyl, 156; heroin, 163; ketamine, 58; LSD, 70; marijuana, 112; methadone, 153; oxycodone, 156; prescribing trend impact on, 1, 2, 138, 169; tranq dope, 148

stroke, 12, 89; bath salts, 42; benzodiazepine withdrawal, 182; cocaine, 190, 196–97; GHB, 66; heroin, 139; ketamine, 57; methamphetamine, 204–5; speedballing, 194

Suboxone, 152

sudden sniffing death, 98

swallow: bath salts, 40; drug packets, body packers, 44; fentanyl, 133; GHB, 64; hallucinogenic mushrooms, 78; hydromorphone, 143; Jell-O shots, 23; LSD, 71; methadone, 151; methamphetamine, 200; oxycodone, 170

sweating, 12, 13; antihistamines, 35; barbiturates, 181; belladonna, 105; cocaine, 195; GHB, 65; hallucinogenic mushrooms, 80;

marijuana, 118; opioid withdrawal, 135, 141, 145, 148, 155, 167; serotonin syndrome, 31

synthetic cannabinoids, 119

syringe, 158; heroin, 141; hydromorphone, 141–44; invention, 156; Jell-O shots, 23; methamphetamine, 201; naloxone, 17; paregoric, 164; shared, 141, 144; speedball, 194

syrup: antihistamine, 34; codeine, 124–26; dextromethorphan (DXM), 87–93; ipecac, 15; Lean, 126–27; methadone, 154; morphine, 160

tea: belladonna, 103, 105–7; caffeine, 185–86; cocaine, 190; fentanyl, 133; kratom, 110–11; mescaline, 84; morphine, 160; peyote, 84; poppy seed, 159, 165–67; Spice/K2, 119, 121, 123

temperature, body, life-threatening, 12, 13; antihistamines, 33, 36; bath salts, 39–41; belladonna, 104; cocaine, 196; dextromethorphan (DXM), 90–91; ecstasy, 52; methamphetamine, 205; rubbing alcohol, 21, 26

thiopental, sodium, 11, 175–76, 183

Tina, 201

tobacco, 40, 59, 121, 140; treatment of addiction to, 75

toke, 116

toot, 192

toxidrome, 6, 9; anticholinergic, 13; hallucinogen, 14; opioid, 10; sedative-hypnotic, 11; stimulant, 12

tranq dope, 40, 130, 132, 135, 148. *See also* xylazine

tremors, 12; barbiturate withdrawal, 181–82; bath salts, 42; caffeine, 188; cocaine, 196; dextromethorphan (DXM), 90; GHB, 65–66; hydromorphone withdrawal, 145; kratom, 109; methadone withdrawal, 155; methamphetamine, 202; prescription stimulants, 211; Spice/K2, 121

trip, 71, 84

tripping balls, 50

trip sitter, 58, 61, 72, 76, 81, 83, 86, 91

truth serum, 91, 173, 175–76

urine, 6; blood-tinged, tainted-Spice/K2, 122

urine, drug screen: false positive for PCP, 88; GHB, 66; methadone, 150; poppy seeds, 157, 160; roofies, 55

MIFFIE SEIDEMAN has called Arizona home for over thirty years with her amazing family. She received her Doctor of Pharmacy from the University of Illinois College of Pharmacy and found her passion in newborn intensive care and drug safety. Miffie spent over two decades in that field and loved training the next generation of pharmacists to care for the tiniest and sickest of babies. She also helped develop a specialized computer nutrition program for premature babies and has been published in peer-reviewed pharmacy journals. She loves using her pharmacy knowledge and career experience to assist other authors through their writing journey. When Miffie is not elbow-deep in drug information, she writes fantasy novels and trains for triathlons.